LET'S TALK ABOUT SEX

ANN-MARLENE HENNING

Let's Talk About Sex

Real Stories from a Therapist's Office

TRANSLATED BY Jamie McIntosh

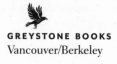

GREYSTONE BOOKS
Vancouver/Berkeley

Greystone Books Ltd.
greystonebooks.com

Cataloguing data available from Library and Archives Canada
ISBN 978-1-77164-428-0 (pbk.)
ISBN 978-1-77164-429-7 (epub)

Editing by Stephanie Fysh
Proofreading by Alison Strobel
Cover design by Nayeli Jimenez
Text design by Belle Wuthrich
Cover photograph by Nele Martensen

Printed and bound in Canada on ancient-forest-friendly paper by Friesens

This work reflects the ideas and opinions of the author. It aims to provide useful information on the
topics covered in these pages. Neither the author nor the publisher is offering medical, health, or
other professional services in this book. Before putting the suggestions in this book into practice or
drawing conclusions from them, readers should consult their general practitioner or another competent health professional. The author and the publisher are not responsible for any liability, damage,
loss, or risk, whether personal or otherwise, suffered as a result of the direct or indirect use or applica-
tion of any element of the contents of this work. Patient names have been changed to protect privacy.

Greystone Books gratefully acknowledges the Musqueam, Squamish, and
Tsleil-Waututh peoples on whose land our office is located.

Greystone Books thanks the Canada Council for the Arts, the British Columbia
Arts Council, the Province of British Columbia through the Book Publishing
Tax Credit, and the Government of Canada for our publishing activities.

Canadä

BRITISH COLUMBIA   BRITISH COLUMBIA
ARTS COUNCIL
An agency of the Province of British Columbia

Canada Council   Conseil des arts
for the Arts   du Canada

Contents

Introduction

A LITTLE WHILE AGO, I gave a lecture on sexuality at a professional development week for orthodontists. Maybe you're asking yourselves, *What on earth does orthodontics have to do with sex?* A lot, actually! The pelvic floor, which spans the area beneath the pelvis, is indispensable for good sex and also works in close alliance with the jaw. Both are part of the human fight-or-flight mechanism, and if someone is being stubborn or for some other reason gritting their teeth, it is highly likely that changes are happening down below, too. It is precisely for this reason that a good sex life leads to so much relaxation—even later, at the office!

I arrived at the orthodontists' event under blue skies and glorious summer temperatures, just in time for the lunch break. The participants, in good humor, were eating on the hotel terrace squinting against the sunshine, or sitting in deck chairs with sea-blue-striped cushions enjoying a post-meal coffee. At small bar tables, others happily chatted away. Once I had loaded my plate and squeezed myself into a place at a table, there was a sudden hush in the conversation—the sexologist had arrived. And there it was, that common tension: "Oh, so now it's all about sex!"

All in all, the week was a success. I was able to communicate my ideas, and the four lectures I gave were well attended. On the first day I asked the participants to take full-length cellphone portraits of their neighbors. What does your body look like? How do you hold yourself? Are you aligned and perpendicular? For the final lecture, I decided to get everybody to end with movement—I wanted us all to sing and dance erotically. But would the orthodontists play along?

I needn't have worried. Ten seconds after I'd started the music, the whole group was on their feet. The participants draped their suit jackets and sweaters over their chair backs and began swinging their pelvises with gusto and singing along with me: "*Ich hab Sex Appeal*"—"I've Got Sex Appeal," a Georg Danzer song. Thirty-seven singing, shimmying orthodontists: a sight for sore eyes—and ears!

It's always a joy to witness how much fun, positive energy sexuality can release. It often begins with giggling that quickly develops into a deep-down belly laugh full of pure life. I try to convey this sense of fun on TV talk shows when I'm demonstrating thrusting techniques, on my vlog when I sit on a table in my socks saying, "Today I'm feeling menopausal," and through my day-to-day work in my practice. People come to me because they want to solve a problem, to learn to speak about their sexual desires, or to reintroduce energy to sex and their relationships. Almost all my clients are surprised about just how much is possible.

Are these things connected to love? Fundamentally, yes. When I'm discussing sex, I like to talk about the "practice of love," because for me love becomes relevant when it's experienced practically and not just talked about. *Practice,* a word with Greek roots, means, among other things, "deed" or "activity" but also "execution," "completion," and "encouragement." It is a word that suits sex well because sex is one of the most important acts for turning love and relationships into reality.

Sadly, whether with a therapist or their partner, many people simply don't dare talk about their sexual acts. It seems to me that we still, or once again, live in an uptight society. Recently a pastor wrote to me that he had covered the subject of "responsible acts in love and partnerships" in a religious education class for sixteen-year-olds. He was immediately suspended from teaching. No nudes were necessary for that step to be taken—a few Bible passages, such as 1 Corinthians 13, and François Villon's raunchy poetry were enough.

I had a similar experience. In 2013 a writ from Germany's Federal Review Board for Media Harmful to Minors arrived in the mail. There was to be a hearing about whether my first book, *Make Love,* a sex education guide for teenagers, was spreading compromising material. Fortunately, I later received an official notice telling me that the matter had been dropped. The whole thing was absurd, because at the same time I had been nominated for a national children's literature award.

In Germany, where I live, official guidelines govern what can be broadcast and when. My TV show can be broadcast in its entirety only after ten o'clock in the evening; the same applies to accessing it on the internet. Apparently, it's easier to accommodate fictional sex and violence on TV than it is to accommodate proper information about sex.

Inhibitions about and blockades put up against the subject of sex also arise in my practice. The media is full of sexual messages and sex is omnipresent in advertising, yet despite this—or maybe because of it—people still haven't got used to a relaxed handling of the subject. A lot of people are ashamed, some so much that I'm reminded of previous centuries. My clients often explain to me how uneasy they feel inside their bodies and with their sexual desires. Only small children are relaxed and natural about their bodies and desires, and for me this is the crux. Sexual attitudes are planted early in people's lives and develop over the years. One of my major concerns is achieving some sort of balance over sexuality from the very start. If parents are relaxed about these issues, then they can also be relaxed about their offspring's sexual and bodily curiosity.

It seems to me that Scandinavians are less inhibited about sex. When I was growing up in Denmark, the subject was pretty much incidental. When we wanted to buy an ice cream at the shop across from my school, we had to pass a porn magazine vending machine right next to the entrance. It was a rectangular box with lots of square glass windows; you placed money in a slot and opened up the flap to take out the magazine. We never did—we didn't have the money for that—but depending on how the shop owner had arranged them, the loosely rolled magazines sometimes offered a clear view of a crotch or a blow job. We didn't find the magazines particularly special; we were indifferent to them. They didn't damage me, and they weren't against the law. Pornographic narratives and images were legalized in Denmark in the '60s, making Denmark the first country in the world to permit them.

With this book, I would like to give you a sense of what it means to be a sexologist and to show you my work with my clients. (Don't worry—you won't recognize your neighbors:

all the people appearing in these pages are disguised to such an extent that they wouldn't even recognize themselves.) I am convinced that the problems, wishes, and sexual desires that clients bring to my practice will be familiar to many readers. I also want to talk about sexuality in a shared language, one that is relaxed and professional with a pinch of humor. I'll not only enthuse about sex but also illustrate ways you can take your sex life to the next level.

People who don't want to talk about sex don't have to. People with problems, however, sometimes do want to seek help and need to learn how to talk about those problems. Sexuality is inherent in us all, and this notion unsettles many of us: shouldn't it mean that things therefore automatically go smoothly in bed? And if things don't work that well for me, could something be fundamentally wrong with me? This is rarely the case as, hopefully, this book will demonstrate. The beauty of life is that one never ceases to learn throughout it, as shown by brain research. And talking to each other helps the process.

1

Symbiosis:

TOO CLOSE
FOR COMFORT

ALMOST ALL MY clients are physically and mentally healthy. They may arrive convinced that something is wrong with them, that they're totally different from other people. They might even have received medical diagnoses that seem to support their doubts. However, they mostly leave their first visit to my office knowing and anticipating that they'll learn something about themselves, and feeling that they're as normal as everybody else. Physically, everything is fine: all that's wrong is their mental perceptions and their lack of knowledge about themselves and their bodies.

An example: A young woman who had never had an orgasm asked me once whether there was anything she could do about not coming. Her problem was most likely hereditary. As an alternative cause, she suggested that she'd "ruined something while riding"—as a child she'd been a keen horseback rider.

First of all, no woman "ruins" her ability to have an orgasm by horseback riding. Just the opposite: riding gives the sex organs a boost through pelvic movement that encourages circulation; in the brain, synaptic paths that are also switched on during sex are energized and boosted.

But women who haven't yet learned to climax often despair. They tell me that they'll be deserted by their partner or will no longer be able to find one because a "certain something" is missing. Many men and women are totally convinced that it's easy and normal to have an orgasm.

A woman who doesn't come can still be rejected as "frigid." She ends up like a broken clock, destined to be stashed in a dark drawer for years . . . but a clockmaker could easily get her ticking again.

Frigid means "sexually cold." The term came into use years ago by doctors who neither understood nor tried to understand female sexuality. I never use the word; it has become obsolete. What exactly is to be understood by it is, in any case, unclear. Inability to have an orgasm? Certainly not. A client once told me, "My girlfriend can't come, she's frigid." On closer questioning, he admitted, "Well, okay, she can come when she does it herself, but never during sex!" I wanted to know what he meant by "sex," and he explained that she normally came with oral sex or fingering but never during "actual" sex. She was simply "frigid." Aha! Evidently, this man considered only vaginal orgasms to be "proper" orgasms—another misconception. Only a small percentage of women come solely from penetrative intercourse. Looking at it from a different angle, in this man's judgment a large percentage of women are frigid.

"Up to now, all the women I've been with have come," he added. Did he realize that, on their own admission, 90 percent of women have pretended to climax at least once?

Incidentally, the man in question had never had a long relationship; he was always the one dumped. I suggested bluntly (I couldn't speak any other way) that he reconsider his ideas about women. Inwardly, I was asking myself whether with such limited ideas he *could* be a good—meaning sensitive—lover and partner.

At least my client had a thoughtful look on his face as he left my practice. Of course, he never returned. From his perspective, *he* wasn't the problem. Sometimes, however, the cause of being uptight really is to be found elsewhere.

One Call Too Many

I REQUIRE CLIENTS to make appointments by email; my assistant, Anika, takes care of the details. Many couples believe they have to prepare me for their problems before the first appointment, as if we need a bit of foreplay. However, the less I know, the more impartial I am at our first meeting and the better I can concentrate on their medical history. So I avoid the telephone.

However, Andrea, who was about to have her initial consultation, called the office shortly beforehand because something urgent had cropped up. I accidentally picked up the receiver, intending to make a call myself.

"Hi, I'm Andrea Schulz," she said. "I've never been to your office—my first appointment was to be next week—but I'm afraid I'll have to cancel it." She had a young voice, though I thought she was probably over thirty. There was uncertainty in her inflection, but not only that—sometimes she sounded as if she was used to issuing orders. I imagined she was a mother. Mothers are always having to explain things to their children, to get them to understand what they're allowed to do and what they're not. As a mother myself, I know the sound of this voice. "Do you have any other appointments free?" she asked. I took a moment too long to answer, so she repeated the question.

"Yes, of course," I replied. "Are you coming alone or with your partner?" I asked this to find out whether we needed a sixty-minute or a ninety-minute appointment. At that very moment I realized that dear old Anika should be taking care of all this, not me!

A short pause. Finally, Andrea said in almost a whisper: "With Harold."

"Harold is your husband, is he?"

"Yes, and the father of our two children. We would like couples therapy." So I wasn't far wrong—Andrea was a mother, of two, in fact. And from the way she said "couples therapy" I had the impression she was giving the words extra emphasis, which said to me that she was not thoroughly convinced about what she was doing at this moment and that she would actually have preferred to cancel the appointment instead of rescheduling it. But somehow she persevered—something was impelling her to follow the path she had already started on.

"Could you contact us again by email?" I asked. "My assistant doesn't like me messing with her appointment calendar!" I laughed. "She's trained me well. Anyway, then we'll have things in writing."

Andrea apologized profusely, although she had done nothing wrong, while I promised myself, and not for the first time, never again to touch the office telephone. All the same, I was curious what this couple was concerned about. Sexuality? Love? Or maybe, as so often, both?

Love and sex: Most people think they belong together—often because they don't want to properly come to terms with the differences between them. To do so would mean dealing with their own personality and their own love and sex lives, and for many people this is not pleasant.

For a long time it was thought that women in particular, almost by their very nature, were unable to separate sex and love. Men, on the other hand, could, which was also given as a reason why, as was assumed to be the case, they were more often unfaithful. This assumption, however, contradicts the facts: women are also unfaithful—and just as often. As far as numbers are concerned, there's no marked difference in this between men and women. So the cliché that women can have sex only when love is involved is also wrong. In my practice I've heard women say countless times, "If only—just once—my husband would just want sex!" These women want nothing other than to get laid, just to get down to business, to screw—with or without love.

"Sweetheart, Can I Tell Ms. Henning?"

AT 7:00 P.M. on the dot, the office doorbell rings: Andrea and Harold have arrived. Andrea is pale, with fresh rouge applied to her cheeks, slim, and average height. Harold is also not a particularly robust type. He's a little less pale than his wife but obviously isn't out in the fresh air with his children as often as some other fathers. I imagine that he does something in IT. I was slightly off on Andrea's age—she is, judging by her wrinkles, probably in her late thirties, so a bit older than she sounded on the phone. Harold, I guess, is in his mid-forties.

I invite them to come in, which they do cautiously, with a quick glance around the large room that opens up before them. Most clients stand there for a while, turning on the spot—symbolic of their situation, as it were. And so it is with Andrea and Harold. I read the astonishment in their faces. They hadn't expected a rose-red velvet sofa with patterned cushions. Ditto the huge painting of three women in a gentle, highly erotic bondage scene. Spread through the room are other posters, on subjects like the pelvic floor or the brain. One wall is covered with bookshelves—my library. Next to it is a large mirror for exercises.

"The red wall is *super!*" says Harold, pointing toward the sofa, which is in front of a wine-red wall. All the other walls are plain beige.

"Do you live here too?" asks Andrea.

I'm always surprised by this question. Okay, my office does feel cozy and personal, but there are no personal things lying around. All in all it's tidy and uncluttered but, apparently, not like a typical office.

"I just want a warm atmosphere so that we feel comfortable," I explain. "After all, we aren't going to be talking about shopping lists here!" Although we do precisely that sometimes, when we discuss lubes or condoms and one or the other gets written down on a list of things to buy.

"Take a seat," I offer. The two identical mauve armchairs seem to literally invite Andrea and Harold to make use of them. The couple, however, remain standing, and I register them both looking at me inquiringly, perfectly synchronized. I begin to wonder whether I have a symbiotic couple in front of me.

"You can sit wherever you like," I add.

Nevertheless, Harold asks, "And where's *your* favorite place to sit, Ms. Henning?"

I laugh. Many clients ask the same question. "I have no favorite place," I say. (However, I have!)

Now this slightly indecisive couple have to make a decision. As I expected, Harold, courteous as a cavalier, now asks Andrea, "Honey, where would you like to sit?"

Andrea answers immediately: "And you, sweetie?" After glancing at me briefly, she adds brightly, "Let's sit on the sofa—it's your favorite, isn't it?"

I grin. Andrea has long since decided where her partner would like to sit—without exchanging words.

"Of course." Harold beams at her. I'm beginning to overheat from all this mutual radiance.

The seating arrangements at the first session can reveal a lot about a couple. Their choices give me a chance to hazard my first cautious conjectures: Are they harmonizing? Do they sit close together, or farther apart? Does a man drop immediately into the armchair or sofa, without making eye contact with his female partner? If so, does she then show her dismay? Would she prefer that he be more gentleman-like, like in an old Rock Hudson or Robert Redford movie? Then he should have sat down only once *she* decided where she would sit. (And if she later has to go to the restroom, then he had better get up politely on her return!) But he didn't. What now? Well, maybe they've got it just right, and he doesn't need to make allowance for her. But then again, maybe he should, as she's already pretty angry with him.

Sometimes both partners stand there helplessly, hesitating. They can't come to a decision and instead await instructions because they really don't want to make any mistakes. Is this what it's like in bed with these two? I'd wager yes. If each is afraid that the other might not like something, then neither will feel like trying something new—it would be like treading on thin ice. Other people do just that and sit wherever they want. Some partners play down their unease with this behavior with offhand remarks: "Okay, then, I'll just sit next to him—it really doesn't matter where we sit, does it?"

All these create impressions that do have to be verified later. But these impressions can often reveal important clues about a couple's love and sex lives.

Harold and Andrea seem to be neither particularly decisive nor particularly indecisive. They seem to be emotionally dependent on each other in a special way, and I will have to be careful that my methods don't encourage this dependence. I want to view the couple as separate people. Only then will it be possible to show them things happening that even they weren't aware of.

Andrea has reached a decision for both of them by choosing to sit on the sofa. Once they've sat down, I can observe how Harold places his hand on Andrea's—a reassuring gesture that Andrea responds to by squeezing his hand in return.

You might think this is a loving couple who are there for each other. But you could also think they're a couple who *need* to hold on to each other. One doesn't have to exclude the other. One important aspect is that throughout the sessions, Harold and Andrea learn to come to a solution, their decisions being arrived at independently and without anxiety about disappointing each other.

Both of them then give some thought as to who will say something first. There's some rattling going on behind their eyes. I can even see little beads of sweat on Harold's forehead. Andrea begins kneading his hand.

"It's great that you came," I start. "I'm sure you find the situation here unusual. I'm a stranger to you ..."

Harold and Andrea nod gratefully.

"Okay," I say. "What do you want to get off your chests?"

Harold turns to his wife. "Would you like to start?" he asks, smoothly and gentlemanlike.

"No," Andrea replies, and then quickly adds in a hushed tone, "I'd rather you start."

Will they feel confident enough to speak openly and honestly in my presence? Will they be able to say something that might hurt the other? Without being able to reassure the other with some form of physical contact? Symbiotic couples have one big problem: if one of them shows some form of independence—for instance, having an opinion that the other doesn't necessarily share—the other becomes insecure. An uneasy feeling creeps in that their partner wishes to move away from the common intimacy and possibly even pull out of the relationship. Anxiety and worry play important roles in our love and sex lives, and I will often return to this emotion of fear. Enough of that for now, but would *you* find someone who is constantly afraid of being abandoned sexy?

The longer I observe Harold and Andrea, the clearer my feeling is that the people sitting on the sofa opposite me are a symbiotic couple. But to begin with, I keep this to myself. My approach is to always be two steps *behind* my clients: they should tell *me* where their problems lie. This way we're on an equal footing.

"We hardly ever have sex anymore," Harold eventually says somewhat mechanically, and Andrea nods. I notice that Harold is about to continue, so I remain silent. He does go on, although he's very careful with his wording: "Both of us just don't feel like it."

"And what do you mean when you say, 'hardly ever have sex'?" I enquire.

"We sleep with each other at the very most once or twice a year."

"How long has this been going on?"

Harold glances at Andrea. "Since the children were born, isn't it? What do you think?"

Andrea nods again. "Yes, after Stella was born. From then on, it was less and less often."

"How old is Stella?" I ask.

"She'll be eight this summer." Their faces show signs of surprise, almost as if they find that difficult to believe.

"A long time," I say, acknowledging their expressions. "But it's nothing unusual," I add to try to comfort them. "It sometimes happens in long-term relationships."

At the beginning of a partnership, when we're in love, our brains release sexual and happiness hormones, such as dopamine, en masse. We get hooked, almost like we're on drugs. We crave our partner's body, and we can't get enough of it. But this isn't a permanent state—unfortunately, you could almost say. Still, nonstop sex is enjoyable only to a point. To put things into perspective: who wants to eat hamburgers every day, even if it's their favorite food?

"But why?" asks Andrea.

"I guess all sorts of things can get in the way," I offer as an initial explanation.

"I can sure agree with that," says Harold. "We have a house with a big yard that needs a lot of attention. We have a long-haired collie, rabbits, two children who also have hobbies ... I have to look after my mother, who will have a go at almost anyone. She's even at odds with Andrea. And Andrea's parents live five hundred miles away and we have to visit them sometimes so the children have some sort of contact with their grandparents." He gasps for breath. I'm pretty certain he could keep extending the list. All these things probably rattle through his head when he's lying in bed next to Andrea at night and wondering why they're no longer intimate.

"When do you have time for each other?" I ask.

They look at me in astonishment, then Andrea answers: "Hardly ever. Everything's planned. Luckily, we usually agree, so at least there are no arguments."

There it is again! Symbiosis. Sometimes couples are missing a necessary ingredient for sex—craving! A craving for something different, so different that it's exciting. For this desire to come into being, you need a counterpart, a person who may not need to be a complete stranger but could be just a bit of one. Then you can explore this strangeness—the adventurer in you is called on. Curiosity is aroused. If you're in love, all this happens naturally, as if of its own accord. But little by little the craving diminishes. Your partner becomes more and more familiar. The strangeness disappears—and with it, desire. Eventually, you become like brother and sister or old friends ... and *not* like passionate lovers.

I catch myself thinking, *If only they'd argue, there would be a bit more friction between them.* But in the long run, arguments aren't what we're looking for in couples therapy.

Suddenly Harold whispers something to his wife: "Sweetheart, can I tell Ms. Henning ...? We don't have to ... but ..."

Harold doesn't need to convince her. Andrea is instantly in favor of his suggestion. "Of course! If you want to, go ahead—tell Ms. Henning."

Her husband seems concerned but at the same time relieved. Without hesitation, Harold announces: "My wife can't come. Something seems to be wrong with her." Andrea looks at the floor sheepishly. "Even with her previous partner," Harold adds.

I immediately consider: Can she *really* not have an orgasm? Or ... (Do you remember?) I nod briefly at Andrea and tell her I'll ask her for her point of view soon but I'd like to stick with Harold's comments, as it was he who raised the subject. I ask Harold, "Why was it important for you to tell me that about your wife?"

"It's perfectly normal," Harold retorts.

"What's normal?" I press while keeping an eye on Andrea. "That women can come, or that a man speaks on his wife's behalf?"

He is surprised by my remark and has to think things over quickly. Eventually he says, "It was intended lovingly."

"Okay, we'll let it be for now," I say. Harold seems to have wanted to protect his wife, but I don't think it makes either of them sexy. "Does your wife know how important this matter is to you?"

Harold hesitates and then says, "I don't want to make her feel insecure."

"Is your wife so weak that she would have trouble taking it?"

That was a thrust to test whether there's any foundation to my suspicions of symbiosis and also to underline for them the images they have of each other. I can tell by looking at Harold that I've landed a blow. The situation becomes clearer: Andrea feels pressured; it's important for her to have an orgasm for her husband. And he has a guilty conscience for demanding something from her. At the same time, of course, he would love to be such a great lover that he could give her a climax. And because this is all so tricky, they both avoided broaching the subject.

I sum things up: "I think you are a very symbiotic couple and have a pretty close idea of what the other thinks about the topic—you're good at reading each other." Both look at me in astonishment, as if I've given away a secret.

"Yes, right from the start we were very close," says Andrea, who seems to have rediscovered her tongue.

"We'll have to talk about it, as it's also possible to be *too* close," I continue, and I persist with Harold. "I'd like to return to the word 'normal.' What is normal for you in sex?"

"That women can come."

"Is that really normal?"

"Isn't it?"

While Harold begins to doubt his certainty, Andrea sits up and swipes the hair out of her face. She's all ears. Apparently a possibility has just opened up, one that could unburden her. She looks like she's just downed an energy drink. I don't want to let the chance to comment on the transformation to her body slip. "You seem different," I say. She laughs bashfully. Anyway, at least she now knows that I haven't lost sight of her even though I'm occupied with her husband. My discussion with Harold isn't finished.

"Many women don't reach a climax," I tell him.

My client looks at me incredulously, and then tries to carefully contradict me.

"Well, hopefully there are a *couple* of women who can." There's a slightly biting undertone to Harold's reply, and in the corner of my eye I notice Andrea suddenly slump.

It's time to turn my attention to her. To me, she isn't the type of woman to come to terms with not having orgasms. I've had enough of *those* women in my office. After a while they're pretty relaxed about it; they don't believe that achieving a climax is an absolute necessity—sex is also good without. They've come to the decision that ultimately they aren't missing anything. Andrea, however, is different: she *really* wants to come.

I turn to her. "Would you like to have an orgasm for your husband because you know that it's important to him? Or for yourself?"

"Personally, it's not so important for me." Well, at least Andrea has a different opinion from her husband, but I'm still not ready to categorize her as a woman happy without orgasms.

I use her opinion as a reason to follow up with Harold, who has shown a clear reaction to her words.

"Is it *especially* important to you that your wife comes?"

Harold hesitates. "Yes, it *is* very important." His voice has adopted a strange and sad note. Then he adds, "But she doesn't want to talk about it . . ."

Aha! At last his feelings are emerging. Andrea is sitting there withdrawn and has adopted the posture of someone who needs protection. Harold's sentiments, however, need to be even plainer, which is why I ask him, "You probably find it easy to come?"

An unequivocal nod.

"And because of this you think most women can come— but not your wife. And you think that if she doesn't want to talk about it, then it's not really that important to her."

Harold remains silent, but inwardly he is struggling. I maintain the silence.

"I'd really like to talk to her about it." And with these words he turns slowly toward his wife.

Andrea looks at him for a moment, then looks away. Harold sighs resignedly.

"Why don't you look at your husband?" I ask Andrea.

It's quiet in the room for a while, and I can hear the evening traffic flowing outside my window. Andrea's eyes have filled with tears, while in Harold's I see a glimpse of satisfaction that conveys something like, *And about time, too!* Then, however, these feelings yield to a mixture of pity, guilt, and admiration—admiration that she can endure her supposed failures being treated so openly here in this room. Harold makes an attempt to calm her down, leaning toward her. I place a finger on my lips as a silent *shush*, to indicate that he should wait a bit.

Andrea then speaks very quietly, almost as if to herself, her hair almost completely covering her delicate face: "I'm so sorry . . . I'm scared of losing you if I don't work something out soon . . . I just don't know how." She gulps. "I'm so ashamed. What if it never works out, no matter what I do?" Tears pour down her cheeks.

I pass her tissues in a pretty patterned container made entirely of fabric. The soft box was given to me as a present by a previous client who shed many tears on the couch during therapy. Andrea takes a tissue, the tears increasing. Her shoulders quake and she wrings the tissue in her hands. Harold is suffering with his wife, wanting to help her in some way or other, which he does by bearing her grief and putting his arms around her. After a while he kisses her hair gently, without saying anything. But these gestures are enough, and she began to calm down.

I tell her, "Women can learn to have an orgasm ... Only in very rare cases is there a neurological cause that makes climaxing impossible—so rare, in fact, that in your case I wouldn't even consider it."

Afterward I wanted to know from Andrea whether she masturbates. After some hesitation, she admits that she suffers from a kind of revulsion. It's unusual for her to feel something "down below," and if she does, she ignores it. She explains that Harold watches porn and has "sex with himself." As she says this, I feel she's now holding something important back, and make a small note in my journal, where I've already jotted down a few key words from our conversation. Andrea says that she's pretty sure Harold watches porn because she can no longer arouse him. In her opinion, this is also why the few times they've had sex together, Harold's erection hasn't been particularly successful. Andrea accepts all the blame—and Harold doesn't contradict her. I tell them I'll come back to this point and that it's important that this doesn't just remain a "fact."

The first session is almost over, and the next problem —erectile dysfunction—is already on the table. I am conscious of how complex Andrea and Harold's story is, but also that this is nothing unusual. At least they've managed to talk about their problems in front of me, even though it was quite an effort for them.

At the end of a session I ask how they both feel.

"Very good, astonishingly," Andrea answers calmly, and this time she doesn't look at her husband for reassurance but simply sits there looking at me.

"I'm happy we've finally got started," says Harold, and the underlying impatience in his voice shows not only me that things have taken much too long to get this far. Andrea immediately starts to squeeze the already crumpled white tissues that had been quite happily resting in her lap. She notices that I've registered this. I manage to suppress my impulse to say something—until next time!

For the next sessions, we arrange for each of them to appear individually. With this arrangement, they can each say what they want without being protective about one another. Some couples therapists only treat pairs. As a sexual therapist, however, I place the sexuality of each individual center stage. Who enjoys talking about their masturbation behavior, first experiences with sex, or deepest sexual desires if their partner is sitting next to them listening closely to everything? All that can happen later; initially, a kind of natural shame is not out of place.

The Fragile Bubble of Symbiosis

IN 2011 I was invited to participate in a philosophical salon at a spa resort, a series of events moderated by the philosopher Robert André. The theme was "Love and Self-Respect." I was an honorary guest and sat on a red hotel sofa in front of an audience of sixty. The host's first question was: "What do you think is the greatest danger to love, Ms. Henning?"

"If you're expecting a long answer, then I'm going to have to disappoint you," I replied. "My answer is short and sweet—fear."

The audience became uneasy and whispers could be heard. There were a couple of louder voices. But in the end they all understood: I meant the fear of another person's reaction.

People who reveal exactly who they are, warts and all, make themselves vulnerable to being rejected by their partners.

When fear governs love—and it often does—it transforms relationships. People keep to themselves things that should actually be spoken. Some remain unsaid, maybe for fear of offending, being rejected, or simply out of wishing to not cause pain, while autonomy or independence (even in the form of having your own opinion) threaten symbiosis, which in turn triggers discomfort. But two people who dare not venture out of their own spaces, who fail to concentrate on their own needs but rather focus on those of their partners, are floating in fragile bubbles: these look beautiful, sometimes are even rainbow-colored, but with the slightest jolt they can burst.

We used to make soap bubbles as kids—for days on end. At some stage we discovered that the biggest, strongest bubbles were made from dish soap and a spoonful of sugar. Carefully, you could even play ball with these sugar bubbles, or stick your finger into them. But then, eventually, they too would burst, and the dazzling magic would disappear.

Symbiotic relationships are those in which couples stick to each other like they're sugarcoated soap bubbles. The cardinal rule: whatever you do, don't rock the boat—always back each other up! This way, you're insulated by fear from breaking up and being alone. People living with such close bonds often tend to have problems because they're no longer able to differentiate well enough between themselves and their partners, unable to see each other as different people but see themselves as a kind of puree. And this always affects sex.

The typical image of symbiosis—indeed, the only one that makes any real sense—is of a mother with child in her arms or, even more pointed, a mother with child in her womb. Mother and unborn child are inseparably connected: if the mother dies, the child dies. If a couple are in a symbiotic relationship, they are always struggling with archaic fears that can be traced back to the infantile mother–child bond. And when I work with couples on partner independence (the proper term is *differentiation*, but more on that later), these fears are activated. This can be a challenge. Nonetheless, I'm convinced that symbiosis in adults, for example, Harold and Andrea, has to be broken to some extent, so that people can experience each other as individual, self-reliant beings with their own needs, yearnings, opinions, dreams, and, yes, even fears—without all the bubbles.

Many couples confuse love with polite behavior. My favorite etiquette advice is a little different: Stop keeping everything to yourself, and stop thinking that your partner can't stand it when you say certain things. Let those things be important enough that you have to say them. Don't treat your partner like a little child. The parent role isn't sexy if the gawky kid is your partner. Trust yourself!

The Devil and Romance

AS I CONTINUED to think about Harold and Andrea, I remembered a story about the Devil written by a Danish author, Tim Ray, that I read when I was studying sexology. It was in the prologue to Ray's wonderfully titled *101 Relationship Myths: How to Stop Them from Sabotaging Your Happiness.* Ray begins his story with the Devil sitting in his boiling hot headquarters staring at the freshly branded words on Hell's office wall:

Objective No. 1: To make as many people as possible as unhappy as possible for as long as possible.

He looks at the words and feels somewhat depressed. Despite all his efforts to screw up the human race, he has to admit that his mission, up to now, has been a failure. People seem perfectly happy: they loaf around on Earth loving themselves and others and generally giving the impression that they're pretty content.

The Devil sighs. He knows he'll have to do something about it, or he'll be transferred or even sacked. He has to make people feel really unhappy.

He tries to pull himself together, and in his moment of need he has a brilliant idea, a really ingenious thought: "A relationship," he says to himself, "is the direct route to Hell." Feverishly the Devil begins to write down his evil plan. He decides that if people are to be really unhappy in a relationship, then there has to be a link to lies. He makes a note: "The Four Lies about Relationships. Lie No. 1: *The love that I seek is outside of me.*'" The Devil hops up and down on his Devil's throne: he envisages a flourishing business soon to be listed on the stock exchange. This business model is simply inspired. Just to give the concept a bit more substance, he formulates Lie No. 2: *"The love that I seek is dependent on another person."*

After the Devil has recorded this, he's impressed with his own creativity, so much so that writes down Lie No. 3: *"I can experience the love that I seek only with one special person."* A broad grin appears on the Devil's face. Internet campaigns flare up in front of his eyes: *"The One and Only,"* and *"The Love of Your Life."* Immediately, and to the tips of his toes, he feels how millions upon millions of people eat their hearts out, feel lonesome, and suffer because they will never be able to satisfy the craving inside them. If love can be experienced only with one single person, how do I find her? What if she's already in a relationship? The Devil chuckles into his fist.

Still, there has to be some icing on the cake. Relationship Lie No. 4: *"It's only true love if the relationship lasts forever."* The Devil slaps his thigh and looks satisfied. "Oh yes! That tops everything!" What a brilliant campaign! There is no better guarantee for unhappiness: If someone isn't in a relationship, then they're unhappy because they believe that you can be happy only inside a relationship. They search like mad for true love and doubt that they will ever find it. Someone who is already in a relationship has to remain in it forever—after all, love is only true in eternity. Those who split up will look back on their old relationship as a failure—after all, true love happens only once in a lifetime. Incidentally, the Devil spreads the rumor that Lie No. 4—eternal love—is God's Honest Truth. Ha! As a publicity campaign, it's a real winner.

And the Devil knows a thing or two about marketing. Hollywood should be there to help out. No other industry in the world would be a better broker than California's finest. Bollywood? Hardly less important—they too should be on his team. And let's not forget television. With these combined forces, it should be easy to subject humanity to the necessary brainwashing. The music industry can help with a couple of sappy love songs; the fashion and cosmetics industries can come on board together with women's magazines picking up on trends. Nothing can go wrong! The Devil rubs his hands together and congratulates himself on his masterly ploy. The next Operation Romance is rolled out. And its success is greater, more mind-blowing, and more complete than the Devil had dared to dream.

So much on the subject of symbiotic love.

There are other varieties of love that take place without the need for symbiosis but that are still just as questionable. Take, for example, couples who bicker like stubborn children, fighting for the right to be right as if trying to get something from Mom or Dad at all costs. During therapy sessions, such couples sometimes try to draw me into their quarrelsome relationships by demanding that I declare my position one way or the other. I don't allow myself to be influenced. When I offer an opinion, it is always of my own free will. Sometimes, however, a partner approaches me directly—like Franz.

The Man Who Didn't Want to Come

FRANZ, A SENIOR physician at a hospital a few hours away, wrote that he wanted to give his wife an appointment with me as a birthday present. Anika, my assistant, answered that I agree to sessions only with people who wish to come personally. However, after quite a bit of to-ing and fro-ing, I consented.

His wife, Helen, turned up alone for the agreed-upon appointment. She was a straw-blond Dane, thirty-six years old, petite, and dressed casually in jeans and a loose-fitting pullover. She sat down in one of the armchairs remarking that she didn't actually know what she was doing here. After a few sentences I was certain that only half of the problem was present. The senior physician wanted to see his wife "healed" although it was obvious that we were dealing with a relationship problem. During the gift session, which we used to get Helen's perspective on things, my impression that it was imperative that her husband be present became firmer. So I told her, "It's nice that you came, but next time I would really like you to bring your husband."

A few weeks later, they both made the long journey to my office. We were just about to sit down when the senior physician—roughly forty, a man of solid stature with broad shoulders in a casual blazer—said to me, "What, specifically, didn't you understand in my email, Ms. Henning?" It was clear that he wasn't expecting an answer. His body language, his facial expression, our eye contact, and the atmosphere in the room all led me to believe that inwardly he was under pressure and wanted to gain the upper hand. Or was he trying to make a little joke? Anyhow, in the hospital he was used to being the boss.

Ultimately, it wasn't so important *what* he had said but *why* he had said it. I had to grasp his motivation. It was quite possible that he was making me responsible for getting him into an unpleasant situation when I refused to have further sessions with his wife alone. I decided to show him that I have noticed his attack.

"You think only your wife has a problem. We may find out today that that's true—but maybe you're wrong," I said, adding with a smile, "No diagnosis over the phone, or from what's inside your trousers." (A thank-you to my ex-husband, an orthopedic surgeon, for this saying, which scans somewhat better in German: *Durch das Telefon und die Hose—keine Diagnose.*) I was so direct because right from the start I wanted to have honest contact, to strive for a true and real relationship, and to make perfectly clear that therapy like this has nothing to do with power struggles. I wanted to work *together* with him and his wife. Once I had finished, the strapping doctor slumped into the armchair and remained silent . . . for now.

Had I really answered his question or become defensive about what I hadn't understood, Franz would have immediately known that I was pretending not to be able to read him to avoid stress and trouble, maybe even out of fear of his impressive appearance or title. From that point on, he wouldn't have taken me seriously; he would have governed the sessions, and I would have had to waste energy regaining ground, if that was even possible. I would have agreed to *his* view of the balance of power, thereby strengthening a certain reality—his own. It was better that I clearly state that I wasn't willing to behave like one of his "subjects" at the hospital, but rather would be his confident, relaxed therapist.

There could have been plenty of other answers to his remark: "Actually, you must be reassured that I have my own mind—after all, you're paying good money for it." Or "I thought you realized that your way of solving problems was somewhat inadequate—otherwise, you wouldn't be here!" Or, even harsher, "Okay, I see that you've come here with guns blazing. People do that if they're angry or scared. Which is it in your case?" With this particular man, I sensed that I would be going too far too soon, and saved remarks like these for later.

A therapist, in every situation with all kinds of clients, has to develop a feeling for this kind of precise timing. How much can this particular person take? Not too much, but also not too little. There's a threshold that's just right to trigger change. In fact, increasingly there are "good" answers that show who I am as a therapist and what I have observed. The best ones, however, are the ones that help clients move forward. What is certain—and this is what was important in this case—is that therapy begins from the very moment the client steps into the office.

2

My Life, My Sex

KNOW BOTH THE relationship patterns I've talked about—
symbiosis and conflict. I have experienced both. In my
first longer relationships I fought for my rights. Later,
once I finally had the courage to relax my defenses a little,
I fell into deep symbiotic bonds that were partly unhealthy.
One in particular was problematic. Up to this day, I've
been working on my relationship patterns and feel that I'm
constantly developing—all the way to a capacity for love
and deep empathy. The most important thing is to remain
myself. When I know who I am, life is more relaxed; I don't
have to fight as much, I can be more discriminating, and it's
easier to cope with closeness to another (beloved) person.
This path began for me many years ago in a Danish village.

In my family, they always said, "One day Ann-Marlene
will be an attorney. The way she argues, she's bound to
study law!" And that's what happened—well, actually, if I'm

being honest, only because the school psychologist fell ill shortly before my appointment for career advice. Nowadays, I would probably spend a few minutes longer pondering such an important life choice. But spontaneous curiosity about something new, together with confidence in myself, has accompanied me throughout life—and neither curiosity nor confidence has yet to let me down. The same combination led me ten years later to psychology.

But that was later. One summer I moved from our little village to the big city to study law—which meant swapping an idyllic duck pond with nearby woods and a beach for honking cars and crowds of humans, though there were plenty of nice old buildings too. Right from the start it was obvious that I didn't want to study law. Salvation came in my second year, in spring 1985, when I got to know Dieter from Hamburg. Not even half a year later I abandoned my studies and moved to Germany to live with him. Dieter and I were even engaged. It was all very romantic! Maybe somewhat *too* romantic, or even symbiotic? In any case, in the elation of falling in love I was prepared to give up everything for him and for our love. It soon became clear, however, that I wouldn't be able to live with Dieter's fits of jealousy. He wanted to have me all to himself. From what I know now, I have to admit this was yet another clear indication of a symbiotic relationship.

In the meantime, I had found work at a Danish bank downtown. My job as Jill of all trades was taken too literally by some fellow employees. Putting it diplomatically, I could have rapidly moved up the ladder. But at twenty-one I was still very shy.

At lunch I would look out over the market square. I often saw photographers doing model shoots. It was the era of supermodels. Extremely pretty girls sashayed to and fro in high heels and short skirts performing ballet movements in front of cameras. Always different girls, always new. When I eventually walked past a shoot, someone stopped me with off-hand words spoken in a friendly way—"Hi there, beautiful!" —and pressed a business card for one of the larger modeling agencies into my hand.

As a model I was an outsider. I looked more like a French woman, and had none of the Claudia Schiffer style that was then in vogue. After four years in the modeling business, it was a welcome, almost longed-for, change when an ex-colleague, after intense discussions about her problems, said casually that I was predestined for . . . psychology! "Yeah, right," I said, frankly not surprised. I only had to hear it once. I had always been interested in people and their motivations. I had often noticed, and my friends had too, that I had a talent for helping friends with their personal or interpersonal problems in all sorts of practical ways. I found it easy to put myself in their shoes, and I got plenty of enjoyment from it.

In 1990 I applied for a coveted position studying psychology at the university, was accepted, and proceeded to focus on clinical neuropsychology, which was at that time a new branch of psychology: physiology, anatomy, cells, synapses, hormones, and the brain. Many of my fellow students found the subject too scientific, but that was the very reason I liked it. It was clear to me then that the mind was nothing without the body, and that the brain governs everything. Body and mind are inextricably connected. I financed my studies by modeling—fashion weeks fell mostly during school breaks. So I was alternately a model and a psychology student, happily enjoying the different roles. I felt privileged, as most of my fellow students had to work nights in bars or weekends in cafés for a fraction of my fees. I was twenty-four, had become "unengaged" to Dieter, and was just about to fall in love with a man who, visually, matched my wildest dreams: tall, slim, muscular, angular, slightly bearded, with wonderfully warm, brown eyes, a straight nose, full lips, and everything else in fine fettle, to put it politely. He was a medical resident, and I had the feeling that he spent every other night at the hospital—and not with me. Nevertheless, we didn't have to reduce our lovemaking by any means and were falling in love. Love indeed followed, and for the first time I had the feeling that I would stay in Germany. We married when I became pregnant (unplanned) with our son. The years that followed were both wonderful and stressful. We had frequent disagreements. We were immature and extremely unyielding. Neither of us was prepared to swallow our pride, so we continued to argue. Looking back, I would say that we were both too young and inexperienced to discuss our problems like adults. We also didn't take the time needed to discover what our differences really were. We were too wrapped up in our careers, in childrearing, and everything connected to it.

Then, in fall 1998, something happened that literally turned my life upside down. My son was five. I was at the thesis-writing stage in my studies when, on a golden fall day at the hairdresser's, I had a sudden attack of flickering in my eyes. On the short drive home I could visualize my son in the passenger seat next to me only as a gray film. Later everything returned to normal. But after a while it happened again, fortunately without any sort of pain. With an uneasy feeling in my stomach—and also as a way of admitting to myself that there was possibly something not quite right in my head—I decided to tell my husband. No, I was absolutely certain something was wrong. If I did nothing, it would probably get worse.

After two days and a routine examination in the CT-scan tube, it was clear: I had at least one large aneurysm in my brain, and I would have to be operated on. There was a high risk that during a plane flight, while exercising, during sex, or even on the toilet, a vein in my head could rupture, causing hemorrhaging. Then things would become critical.

To make things worse, during prep for surgery, doctors discovered two more aneurysms. The surgeon said, "I hope we can get all three in one operation." Luckily, they did— but it took seven hours.

After the operation the hardest time of my life began. The surgical intervention was a great success, but I learned that I was pregnant. An abortion was unavoidable, as the postoperative drugs I had to take for three months were dangerous for fetuses in early stages of pregnancy.

Shortly after the abortion, I was once more in the hospital suffering from dizzy spells and speech and visual disorders—a suspected stroke. I was scared, and felt completely helpless. My body was stuck with tubes and needles. It was a terrible experience, as I was no longer getting any information at all about what they were doing to me. Then all of a sudden my whole body was covered in red spots and my lips swelled up like a sex organ. The reason? An allergic reaction to one of the many pills I had to take. On the third day I asked if they had any drugs to help with fear—and was given some without any problems. The fear disappeared and, surprisingly, so did the neurological symptoms that were the reason I'd been admitted to hospital in the first place. It soon became apparent that I was suffering from an anxiety disorder that had probably been triggered by the operation.

So I was discharged from the hospital and dependent on lorazepam, an anti-anxiety drug. I managed, however, to do without the medication by gradually reducing the dosage on my own. But it was awful. The lower the dosage, the more anxiety attacks I had to endure. For one long year I underwent therapy, and finally things returned to normal.

I began to think about my life and realized that during these difficult times I felt emotionally abandoned. Not everyone can withstand always being there for their partner during a dangerous illness. The best thing about the whole affair was that I now knew that I would have to rely on my own strength, and I felt deep gratitude just to be alive. The operation had made it clear that the rest of my life was a finite unit of time, and even though I was just thirty, that life wouldn't last forever. Death had been close, and I asked myself, "Do you really want to continue living like you have been the last couple of years?" I didn't have to think long about the answer: "Definitely not!" So I decided to make the most of my life. I wasn't sure yet what all that would involve.

Childhood on the Move

IN MY EARLY childhood I generally felt as happy as could be. This was not the case later. The reasons for this, I discovered after many post-illness psychology sessions, were the circumstances triggered by my parents' divorce. My father disappeared from my life overnight. He had met another woman.

I had always witnessed my parents as sexual beings. I'd often seen them kiss and hug or give each other a playful slap on the bum. When I was younger, I'd thought that it had been the sex with other women that made my father leave his family, that he was pretty immature for his age. When he later remarried and I ended up with two new half-siblings, I was no longer so sure. But it is cute the way kids think of their parents as always being old. During my therapy, my psychologist, Dr. Timm, and I calculated that my father wasn't forty when he left the family, as I had always believed, but only in his mid-twenties. Since then I've viewed the events of that time differently.

In the four years after my parents separated, my mother, my brother, and I moved house three times. For me that always meant new neighborhoods and schools. Each time I had to stand in front of a class of thirty schoolkids all staring at me. Behind me, my mother would stand with her hands on my shoulders, and behind her, the school principal. Teachers liked me because I did my homework and was obedient, but to the other children I was always "the new girl."

All in all it was a terrible time. I was never invited to parties and had hardly any friends. I was a late bloomer sexually—although I discovered early how to get plenty of good orgasms. But the sad truth was that while my brother, Brian, who was two years younger than me, was kissing girls behind closed doors, I was only imagining all this new and very interesting "body stuff." Admittedly, some twentysome-things and, yes, even older men, wanted me, particularly when they were under the influence of alcohol. But I found them repellent. In a nutshell, during my early teens I would have loved just to dig a deep hole and jump in.

These experiences help me to this day, as many people who come to my practice feel like they're different from other people, that they don't belong, and think they can't do things that others master with ease. I can then say, "I know the feeling." Clients believe me, as they can see it in my eyes—a certain sadness about the fact that my adolescence was as it was and will remain the way it was for the rest of my life.

In 1980 I finally made it to high school. This entailed traveling every day from the countryside to the nearest larger town. The nicest thing about this arrangement was that no one knew me there. I was fifteen and planned to reinvent myself—purely an intellectual decision. I would never be alone again, never be an outsider.

Nobody in high school noticed that up until then I had been an outsider. Slowly, at last, sex became a topic of conversation. It certainly felt as if my girlfriends and I were soon talking about nothing else. Finally I too had a proper boyfriend, Anders. We had sex for the first time when I was almost seventeen. He was two years older and it was also his first time. Playfully, and in a relaxed way, we discovered our sexuality. It was a beautiful and loving relationship until two or three years later. We were living in the big city together when I had an affair with a law student two years older. I was curious and interested in men and just wanted to broaden my experiences, so I split up with my high school boyfriend.

With Alice in Wonderland

I MOVED INTO a shared apartment with Louise, a fellow law student. It was a perfect singles' life. We went out a lot—dancing, dressing up—and had a lot of fun man-watching.

We lived right behind the train station downtown. Sex in the city—and not a duck pond in sight!

For two years I was able to freely experience my sexuality, met many men, and relished everything except my law studies, which I was enjoying less and less.

Socially, I was busy, especially with my oldest friend, Alice. She had been brought up in a strict religious family, which even back then was very unusual in Denmark. When we were children, she lived on the same street as me, and whenever her parents allowed it, we played together. This always had to be planned well in advance, as Alice had a lot of chores to do—cleaning the windows, baking cakes, and then on to a Girl Guides meeting or some sort of evening event at church. She was powerfully yoked, and only after she'd finished everything else could we play. We had fun together and laughed our heads off when we played horsy with our rolled-up bedspreads and felt a certain *something* down below. We squealed *oohs* and *aahs* and made totally crazy faces. We liked it a lot, but somehow we knew that "it" must be forbidden simply because it was so nice. So much pleasure was definitely not intended in Alice's childhood home.

I remember that Alice once asked her stepmother, when she was packing for a school outing, what tampons were. The word was on the checklist of things she was required to pack. Alice's stepmother answered testily, "You don't need to worry about those yet!" And that was the end of that. When Alice, a short while later, had her first period, she was horrified and thought she was going to bleed to death.

At school too sex education was as good as nonexistent. There was one single hour with Mrs. Nunann, my childhood favorite teacher, and that was it. She was about to retire and had nothing whatsoever to do with sex. We giggled nonstop without really listening as she explained falteringly the structure of the sexual organs and how fertilization worked. It was an embarrassing affair.

Others in our small village were more relaxed about sex. My friend Gitte's father, for example, had a subscription to a men's magazine, which he kept on a low shelf in the living room. When Gitte's mother was out, we would leaf though the magazines. We must have been about nine or ten. It was with Gitte that I first played "doctors and nurses" (this was before my "horsy" games with Alice). We made a cozy cave out of blankets, closed the door, and stripped off below the waist. We then rubbed each other's vulvas with the longish and slightly rounded-off head of a Pez candy dispenser and burst into laughter. Then we'd try another dispenser and repeat. But it wasn't only funny—I can distinctly remember the tingle of excitement.

Basically, I always had a soft spot for sexuality. Even back then I was dreaming up dumb ideas! For instance, in order to fool kids in a different class, a friend and I filled small homemade bags with mineral salts and told everyone it was a miracle powder which, when mixed with water, would make their bosoms grow at an amazing rate. Then we disappeared to the restrooms, supposedly to drink the magic potion. While there, we stuffed socks under our shirts and finally strutted around the schoolyard with our newly grown "bosoms." The beauty of it was that everyone believed us.

As was to be expected, Alice didn't have it easy during puberty. Only when she finally moved out did she reach top form. She did as she pleased, neglected her studies, drank a bit too much, and got acquainted with one man after the other. During this phase she often visited me in the city.

It was at this time that Dieter from Hamburg entered my life and we fell in love. One time Alice came to visit when Dieter was there, on a Good Friday.

It was evening. We'd all had something to drink and all of a sudden Alice started to dance. She said that she would now perform a "funny" kind of striptease, which she then proceeded to do. I secretly admired Alice for daring to dance in front of us—I was too shy to even think about it. Alice, in her own way, was also shy, but she was able to cover it up skillfully. She stopped stripping when she was down to her panties, and as she sat down on the bed where Dieter and I were snugly stretched out, the conversation, for some inexplicable reason, turned to oral sex. Who knows how on earth we landed there! Alice said she was pretty good at it. I looked at my happy but somewhat sheepish friend and said, "Try it out on Dieter and show me how." Alice replied, "Can I? Should I?"

I asked Dieter: "She can, can't she?" We laughed a bit uncertainly, but didn't find the idea too awful. The result was that Alice taught me how to give head on my own boyfriend.

Later, thinking about Alice, I was amazed that a person who grew up in a household without sexuality, hostile even to sensuality, could have so much passion for life and get such pleasure from sexuality, while others from far more liberal environments grow up with hardly any need for sexuality and would rather live life without sex at all. How does that happen? What determines people's sexual personality?

The Pleasure Pedal

TO PUT IT another way, where exactly does sexual desire come from? For a long time people seeking answers to this were groping in the dark. And when answer are lacking, hunches are acted on and pills prescribed. Helen Singer Kaplan, a Viennese sex therapist who later lived in New York, believed that there were three phases to human sexual response: desire, arousal, and orgasm. But her approach could not explain how sexual desire works in general. This became possible at the end of the '90s with the dual control model developed by John Bancroft and Erick Janssen at the Kinsey Institute in Bloomington, Indiana. The dual control model is as simple as it is ingenious. It's based on the idea that a central mechanism regulates sexual arousal—how and when someone reacts to sexually relevant stimuli (appearances, smells, feelings, fantasies) or doesn't react.

Bancroft and Janssen allegorized their model as a gas pedal and brake system. The gas pedal represents the sympathetic parts of the autonomic nervous system, and the brakes represent the parasympathetic parts. According to Bancroft and Janssen, desire and arousal are the result of two synchronized processes: stepping on the gas and releasing the brakes. (Normally, the brakes are on. Otherwise, people would be horny all the time—at business meetings, the dentist ...)

People with sensitive brakes are less likely to become engaged in sex; maybe they need a special occasion to develop desire and get started. People who always have their foot on the gas pedal, on the other hand, are easily aroused and can engage in spontaneous sex. Such people find it easy to be sexually active. To put it another way, the gas pedal turns you on; the brake pedal turns you off. How the two systems are tuned in a given person and how sensitively that person reacts to stimulation remains more or less constant throughout life, like other traits that determine personality. The major advantage of the dual control model is that it shows that the braking system and the gas pedal systems depend on each other but, as I've said, run simultaneously and independently.

For example: If during sex a partner says they don't want to do what is at that moment expected of them, desire is rapidly affected. *How* rapidly depends on the tuning of the gas and brake pedals. For someone with a steady gas pedal, a rebuff like that will not have much effect. But for someone with sensitive brakes, it could mean the end of this round of sex. By the way, sensitive brake pedals—regardless of the gas pedal—seem to be the main cause of sexual problems.

Alice and I both have well-adjusted gas pedals; our brakes, on the other hand, are pretty loose. With more sensitive brakes and without an extra gas function as a counterbalance, Alice's strict upbringing would have had an even greater (negative) influence on her love life. My similar system made me sexually open and curious, and with its help I have had many thrilling sexual adventures. For readers who wish to know more, the sex educator Emily Nagoski describes the control model thoroughly in her book *Come as You Are*, which includes a small questionnaire everyone can use to work out their own configurations.

Six turbulent years after my brain operation, I made one of the most important decisions of my life and got a divorce. I split up with the father of my child a good fifteen years after our first kiss. I hardly dare say it, but I was unfaithful to him and already had my next partner on the starting block.

Despite its difficulties, the end of this long and wonderful relationship is a prime example of how many long-term couples refuse to do what must be done: talking honestly to each other. Instead, one partner—in this case, me—decides to take a shortcut out of the relationship by looking for someone else and falling in love with them. I had such longing for intimacy, good conversations, and fun in life that I accepted hurting someone I still loved: my husband. The guilty conscience that could have acted as a brake was hidden by my being in love.

After we separated, I moved into a new apartment just blocks from our previous one. Initially, our son lived alternately with his father and with me, but little by little the eleven-year-old spent more and more time with his father. One of the most difficult things I had to do in life up until then was, at some point, to let him go. It almost broke my heart. Sometimes, even today, I ask myself whether I was wrong. I'm very grateful that when my son has problems, he comes to me, day or night—if anything needs mending, it's Mom's job, as it's supposed to be.

After the divorce I had plenty of time to myself. I was fine. I was still earning money as a model, but the offers were gradually becoming fewer. Then I discovered a new talent. Together with a number of my fellow models, I began singing at fashion shows and other events. We were the Glittergirls. All coiffured and in beautiful evening gowns, we sang close-harmony songs like the Andrews Sisters' "Mister Sandman." At the same time I was taking singing and acting lessons and emceeing events. Everything was okay considered individually, but it wasn't what I actually wanted to be doing. Something had to happen. And then it did!

My best friend in Germany at the time was a translator for the Danish railway company, and often had to travel to Copenhagen, in Denmark. One day, I was once again telling her all my woes over the phone, when she said, "Ann-Marlene, why don't you become a sexologist?"

"Eh?" I said. I was so surprised by her question that I was lost for words.

"Late yesterday," she said, "when I was fetching the key for my office, there was a note on the door. *Please get the key from the sexologists on the next floor.* Up there was a bunch of women just like you." The women my friend was talking about were between forty and sixty. Nurses, psychologists, sociologists, health educators, midwives . . . and they were all studying sexology!

Suddenly it clicked. For years I'd been watching sexology shows on a Scandinavian TV channel. In one show, adults sat in a classroom for sex ed lessons—it was funny. The show was hosted by my future supervisor, Joan Ørting. The British *Sex Education Show* was broadcast on the same channel. German television at that time had nothing like it.

That very same day I applied to the private sexology school in Copenhagen. I was accepted. The teachers were experienced therapists with a variety of specialties, but also sex workers, transgender people, or people with fetishes, among others, who had a chance to present their particular take on things. We also visited a tantra institute and a sex shop and had a whole day of lessons on the scope of various forms of pornography, simply so that we could later be less judgmental in our dealings with clients.

As the curriculum consisted mostly of psychological and sexual practices, as opposed to anatomical or physiological aspects, I later studied a clinical therapy approach that focuses on the body and enables the ability to describe any person's sexual systems. This makes it a highly efficient tool for therapy. The concept features four spheres, each representing a different aspect of sexuality and their interactions—but more on that later.

In spring 2007, I was finally ready: I opened my own sexual therapy practice in my apartment back in Hamburg.

3

Looking Closely in Sex Therapy

W HEN I WAS thinking up a name for my practice, I tried to avoid the usual stereotypes. I definitely didn't want the name to support the widespread belief that participating in couples or sex therapy prepared a client to be a dream partner for life. The words *sex* and *love* shouldn't be part of the name. I didn't want anything esoteric —no fuss, just the basics: I am a therapist for sexuality.

In the end I chose *Doch-Noch,* which translates to something along the lines of "Yes, You Can." The name is meant to suggest an attitude. If someone says to me "It's not going to work—I've tried so much already, but I just can't do it," my reply almost always is: "Are you sure? Perhaps you can!" With this attitude, far more is possible than was previously thought—including where love is concerned. There is almost always hope; very little is set in stone—though the ancient loving, kissing couple depicted between the *Doch* and the *Noch* of my logo very much are.

In Vitlycke, in southern Sweden, just over sixty miles as the crow flies from my native Denmark, tiny little figures were carved into flat rocks during the Bronze Age, and they are very definitely living out their desires. I was fascinated that even long before our times people felt the need to express their sexuality (and love), if only on a stone wall. The ancient loving, kissing couple embody this.

First Impressions

THE STAIRWELL TO that first office in my apartment was extremely dark. Energy-saving bulbs gave off a dim, dreary light when switched on and took an eternity to reach their full glory. After new clients rang the doorbell and I let them in, they had to clamber up steep stairs in this half-light. There were advantages to this for me as a therapist, however, as I was able to observe them undetected and get a first impression.

My present office is on the ground floor and is bright and friendly. Nevertheless, here too first impressions are made, in all the valuable seconds when we first set eyes on each other. Afterward those impressions I gather more detail—but then we're getting into the realm of second impressions. For the first impression of a client, I look at their face, their masculinity or femininity and how these are expressed. Of course, most of the time (but not always!) I can tell whether the client is a man or a woman. But

I also register how masculine or feminine someone acts irrespective of biological gender. Do they cross their legs when they sit, or do they sit with legs splayed? But also: Do they have long hair or short? Do they wear makeup? Over time, though, these details have come to have less and less relevance to gender. Women or men sit this way or that, go seldom to the hairdresser or regularly, and adorn themselves with accessories or not. The fact is, everybody has a male side and a female side, and I'm interested in how this is manifested, as it naturally has a lot to do with sexuality. This is why I take a good look, as objectively as possible, at the person opposite me and how they express their gender—and, almost more importantly, whether they are conscious of this. Are they playing with it? Are they proud of it? Do they (men or women!) favor plunging necklines, or is everything covered up? Is that XL T-shirt or blouse hiding their gender like camouflage? Are they showing off their figure, their muscles?

I pay attention to physiognomy, body language, and facial expressions. Is someone particularly large, small, fat, or skinny? Is that a smile on their face, or do the corners of their mouth tend to point downward? Does a certain expression appear particularly often, and does it betray something about their experiences in life? And what's their body tension like? Their posture? Are they centered and aligned, or do they have hunched shoulders, slouching or sticking their chest too far out? How is their pelvic floor placed relative to this line?

The fact is, how someone carries themselves influences their mood. The body and mind form a unit and influence each other. A person who always stoops doesn't go through life open-minded or radiant but, as their stance implies, rather withdrawn or introverted. People like this probably build some kind of psychological firewall and because of this are less likely to be noticed by others. And maybe that is precisely what they subconsciously mean to achieve!

At this point during my lectures I sometimes use a *Peanuts* comic strip. Charlie Brown is standing there, feeling blue, staring at the ground, his arms hanging lifelessly at his side.

"THIS IS MY 'DEPRESSED STANCE,'" he says. Patty, the cute girl with the pageboy haircut, is behind but says nothing. "WHEN YOU'RE DEPRESSED, IT MAKES A LOT OF DIFFERENCE HOW YOU STAND ..."

Patty listens attentively while Charlie half turns to her and continues: "THE WORST THING YOU CAN DO IS STRAIGHTEN UP AND HOLD YOUR HEAD HIGH BECAUSE THEN YOU'LL START TO FEEL BETTER ..." Charlie turns away again and with his head sagging says, "IF YOU'RE GOING TO GET ANY JOY OUT OF BEING DEPRESSED, YOU'VE GOT TO STAND LIKE THIS." And he is back to his stance in the first frame.

You couldn't describe what the body's bearing does to our thoughts and feelings any better than that. And it works the other way around, too.

The Body Speaks

BIT BY BIT I get a fuller picture of my clients from these impressions. During our conversations I keep an eye on whether and especially when their body language changes. What topics cause frown lines to appear on their foreheads? Are their elbows crossed? Does their body abruptly straighten when previously it was casually leaning back on the cushions?

"Have you noticed that whenever your husband talks about being unfaithful ten years ago, you jiggle your leg?"

"No, I haven't!"

During arguments about stressful subjects, body tension often increases. I then suggest that we try to solve this by discovering the cause.

It's also interesting to notice how close a client is drawn toward me—or if there is movement away from me. The sofa and two armchairs are in specially selected places in my practice, in perfect balance, so that nothing should need to be moved around, but some clients do precisely that. Sometimes it's easier to move a chair than themselves.

I use a little journal to record my observations during a session and make note of key words. I take notes in pencil and later underline in three different colors—green, blue, and red—as a kind of memory jogger for myself.

Green means a topic I wish to return to was discussed or implied. I don't like interrupting and stopping the flow of words, especially when clients are going flat out, as long as they're supplying important information. Red marks obligatory homework (look each other in the eyes for five minutes twice a week, try some frenching, begin masturbating, etc.) to follow up on at the next meeting. Blue means knowledge gained, including "aha" insights that may be relevant at later therapy sessions.

Of course I'm not writing the whole time, just noting key information and important pointers. It doesn't seem to disturb my clients. Some of them are even curious.

"Well? Are you writing something exciting about me?"

"You'd really like to know, wouldn't you," I reply.

"You've probably just written that I'm beyond saving."

"No, no, just a second!" I start leafing back in my notebook. "Here it is: *Increased tension when talking about his ex.*" Maybe it's true, maybe I made it up. "What do you think of that?"

Speaking of pencils, it's been shown in many scientific studies that there is a close connection between facial expression and feelings. In one study, the test subjects were split into two groups (trial and control) and told to learn pairs of words by heart. It's been known for some time that people learn better if they're in a good mood. The control group learned their pairs of words (lemon–Christmas, apple–man, etc.) under normal conditions. The people in the test group, on the other hand, had to grip a pencil with their teeth while learning. Why? Thanks to the pencil, the corners of the mouth are in the "up" position, activating the group of muscles that the brain associates with laughing—so, good mood. Try it while playing a memory game with your partner. They'll be amazed when you win, just like you said you would.

Readjustments

WHEN I WAS thirty-six, I got braces. Ten years earlier my dentist had pointed out that my teeth were misaligned. This misalignment was now responsible for my incisors being forced forward, and the hissing I made with *sh* and *s* sounds could no longer be blamed on having Danish as a first language.

The procedure was more complicated than I imagined. First I was given a bracket to loosen the teeth. When they were loose enough to comically wobble back and forth, it was time for the "styling," and I was given a clamp-like apparatus to keep the teeth in the correct position. At the very end, an operation firmly set the position of the jaw. In total the realignment took two years.

In some respects the procedure reminds me of therapy: in our conversations, my questions ease my clients away from their entrenched ideas. I break down structures, bringing turbulence into their lives—but only for a while. Later the thinking, concepts, and behavioral patterns are readjusted. Another thing I found interesting was that the transformations to my physicality (the loose teeth) affected me psychologically. I felt insecure in a way I had never known before. Everyone around me, whether in my private sphere or people I met when I was out shopping, seemed to realize this. I know because I was treated differently than usual—less politely, more provokingly. I was often snubbed. As a whole it made sense: a person with loose teeth can't attack and can't defend themselves. I was beset by weaknesses, and people who needed to could take advantage of me. Now they could snap at me without fear of being bitten back.

But how did these people know about my weakness? The answer is mind mapping.

Reading Others

OUR BRAINS ARE constantly producing mental pictures of what the people around us think, know, believe, and feel—how they're doing, what they want, and what they will do next to get it. Neuroscientists call this ability *mind mapping*. This has nothing to do with clairvoyance but rather is based on a mixture of experience, anticipation, and self-preservation. And it also applies, of course, to how we perceive our partners. We "read" gestures, expressions, and behavior: not only what is said but, just as importantly, what is left unsaid. All of this is taken in and interpreted, and to a certain degree our own conduct is based on our analysis. Why has my partner been so quiet recently? Is a secret being withheld? If yes, why? Could it harm me or cause me pain? What can I do to protect myself? But also: What are they smiling about? Do they fancy me? Our ability at mind mapping is hereditary and firmly linked to the brain. Mind mapping happens all by itself, all the time, and everywhere—we are all reading each other.

Mind mapping is often confused with empathy, but they have nothing to do with one another. It has been shown that psychopaths and sociopaths feel no pity or empathy for others but are still brilliant mind mappers, able not only to read others but to manipulate them as well.

There is another process in our brains that runs parallel to mind mapping: *masking*. Masking serves to repel attempts by others to mind map by blocking them, keeping your cards close to your chest, and maybe even laying a few false trails. Unfaithful partners sometimes perfect this technique. Not only do they mask, they plant fake realities in their partners' minds, which is also an important component of mind mapping.

All this might sound strategic, egotistical, or even immoral, but it is human. It's hereditary; there's nothing we can do about it. It's also equally pronounced in males and females. Even babies are able mind mappers—albeit in a rudimentary form: they can "read" their caregivers. Are their caregivers happy or sad? Are they frightened? At about four, children can talk about how their parents are feeling.

The less favorable the milieu a child grows up in, the better their innate ability to mind map develops. An insecure background (for instance, a dysfunctional family) has to be particularly and carefully "read" for protection purposes. For some children, this can be about survival. Then the actual ancient function of mind mapping becomes apparent: it increases the chances of survival. But even in healthy families, mind mapping is important for children. For instance, a child with brothers or sisters "reads" more precisely because of the competition—the person who has the best chances of getting out of an awkward situation is the one who recognizes that situation first.

Parents often believe that children don't notice their relationship problems, and here they are almost always wrong. I always try to encourage parents to talk to their children, about, for example, a pending and unavoidable split. Afterward I often get feedback about how their offspring casually explain that they've known the score for a long time. Why were the children so relaxed about it? They were calm because they could rely on their perceptions.

Incidentally, parents gain valuable clues about their children's mind-mapping abilities when they start lying to them. This means that the child has learned to read their parents perfectly, as only when someone has an idea of what the other wants to hear can they lie to them.

Mind mapping naturally plays an important role in a couple's relationship, as it defines the image a person has of their partner and also how that person behaves toward them. In therapy, highlighting these images and establishing mind mapping as a tool can be enormously useful.

A woman says, "I'm just trying to be helpful when I tell him what to do."

Her husband frowns.

"What do you think your husband thinks about what

you've just said?" I ask. Even though she's seen his reaction, she claims to have no idea.

"And if you *did* know?" I probe. She remains silent and pretends not to be able to read him.

So I turn to the husband. "Your wife says that she's trying to be helpful when she bosses you around. How does this make sense when she knows you don't like it?"

"Maybe she doesn't care," he replies cautiously before hitting the nail on the head: "She isn't trying to be helpful—she knows exactly what she is doing!"

Now it's clear why the man frowned—it was a physical reaction to his wife's lie. He knew the real motivation because he had mapped her. I tell him this and now he is aware: she's not being helpful; she wants control.

Mind mapping is authentic relationship communication that happens right in front of us and in real time. It is brain-to-brain linking. Couples behave like a well-oiled machine, but sometimes one partner claims to not be able to read the other. Often they pretend not to recognize why a partner behaves the way they do in order to avoid unpleasant truths in their relationship. Relationship problems are considerably easier to dodge if we convince ourselves that our partner had no idea they were causing pain by behaving in this way or that. When a person who is very close to us hurts us, we prefer to believe that it was unintentional, or that they were being stupid or naive. If they knew what they were doing, well, that would be mean or cruel. The bitter truth is, they do, in fact, know it. Almost always. If we were to admit this, we would have to discuss it—and might even have to split up if the behavior continues. It is precisely this that causes us to shy away from delving deeper.

The realization that a partner can sometimes be mean or egotistical can be very important to couples. So too can accepting that both partners generally know far more about each other than they are prepared to admit, that they mask things from each other, and sometimes even try to project a false self-image.

Knowledge of our mind-mapping capabilities means that partners can no longer hide behind comments like "Oh, I didn't realize I was irritating my partner." Instead they begin to take on responsibility for themselves and their relationship.

After therapy, couples should be able to look at each other using their good side and not their bad one. They can then talk about their "readings" calmly. I often explain mind mapping as a kind of "reading" that allows feelings, moods, and motivation to be understood in order to gain information. More about that later.

This is why I try to make every couple aware that they really do read each other—precisely and accurately. Once they have understood this, we can use this "fact" in therapy sessions. The conversations gather momentum, and so does the development of the couple's relationship.

Who's Mapping Whom?

CLIENTS ARE, NATURALLY, mapping not only their partners but also their therapists—in general even faster than therapists are reading *them*, as clients are being instinctively vigilant. As a result, I have to be careful. If I use overly direct, aggressive questions to glance behind clients' facades, to crack structures—in short, to unmask them—their internal alarm may start ringing, and they will clamp shut like oysters. Too much caution, however, is just as undesirable. Clients will also map this, and possibly use it to cleverly bypass unpleasant topics.

A responsible therapist is continually becoming familiar with their *own* patterns and weaknesses, as clients know when they're being fooled. Basically, a therapist can bring a client only as far as the point of maturity that the therapist has already reached themselves.

Another fact is very important to me: clients paint a picture of themselves as they would like to be seen. They know that during therapy they will be carefully observed, and they want to appear in the best light. If I accept these images without challenging them, they become the truth. I'm not then actually helping my client, even though they might feel reassured. But clients are here to change their reality, which is why my attention is particularly on the dark corners of the pictures, on the things left unsaid, the flaws, and the inconsistencies. These point the way to the core of the problem.

4

Passion Crash:

WHEN MEN'S EQUIPMENT LETS THEM DOWN

ALMOST EVERYONE WHO comes for their first appointment in my office is nervous. People wonder a lot (too much) about how things are going to turn out, and think, *A psychologist looks at my psyche—what on earth is a sexologist going to look at? Yes, exactly! My bed or, figuratively, at least, my underwear!*

Clients usually imagine a given procedure, as if there are rules of some sort about how things happen in therapy. But how to begin and then proceed, as well as what I do exactly with my clients, is decided *during* the first session. There are no fixed rules, no rigid patterns.

You could assume that with topics like sex the majority of clients would arrive alone, as the subject is a bit delicate, but in fact many come as couples. Actually, that should be obvious, as couples therapy and sex therapy are closely linked. Something that isn't right in the relationship has an effect on sex, and vice versa. Cause and effect are difficult to differentiate—just as they were for Harold and Andrea. Remember those two?

Dropping Your Pants

HAROLD ARRIVES TEN minutes late for his individual session. He's been held up by traffic. But he is aglow with anticipation of soon being free to talk about his biggest problem without his wife, without having to take her feelings into consideration. He's in a very good mood. Will this soon change? My plan for the day is to cover more issues than he's probably bargained for.

As he takes a seat on the sofa, I ask him how he's been since the last appointment. "Really well."

"And your wife?"

"She was sad, but somehow more relaxed than normal. In the evening we even kissed and almost had sex..."

"How did that happen?"

"It was weird...She cuddled up to me in bed and then things happened almost automatically."

"Almost?"

"Yes...My equipment let me down. Just as things were about to heat up, my erection as good as gone." He speaks softly. "The final blow was the condom."

"You use condoms?"

"My wife doesn't want to take birth-control hormones."

"What happened then?"

"It was fine—we slept with our arms around each other."

He seems honest enough, but I imagine a little, conspiring voice deep in his subconscious saying to him, "Okay, it was fun, but what if this continues? It's bound to happen again!" And already we've landed in the realm of erection difficulties. I'm sure that we'll also get around to the consumption of porn—after all, I saw the guilty look on Harold's face when Andrea mentioned how he'd developed a habit of watching porn and wanted sex with her only occasionally.

It's completely normal that a man his age has a softer erection than in his youth, but depending on the quality of the arousal, various problems can arise with age.

Two questions are immediately on the tip of my tongue. First, how much pressure is on Harold—both physically and mentally? And, second, how exactly does he arouse himself?

"So, the problems with the erection: when was the first time it happened? Your wife has already broached the subject."

"I don't know. It only happens when I want to have sex with her. When I do it myself everything's fine."

"Can you describe it in a bit more detail? When *don't* you have problems?"

"Well, when I masturbate. To porn clips."

"And how often do you do that?"

"It's become more frequent. When we were still having sex, once a week. But since we no longer sleep together, well, actually every day. Always just before I go to bed."

I nod and Harold continues as if he really wants to unburden himself.

"My wife goes to bed before me—I have to take the dog out. Usually Andrea is still reading when I return. On the way home I use the bathroom in an outbuilding on our property and find one of my sites on my iPad. Then I get down to business very quickly."

"What do you mean by 'very quickly'?" I ask this question because it's important to know how long someone takes to reach a climax. From this you can learn how much enjoyment they could possibly get from that particular form of arousal. Those who are quick barely have time for arousal. The end result—the climax—isn't a particularly satisfying event. On the other hand, more time tends to lead to more quality.

"Two, three minutes . . . maybe." Harold looks gloomy, as if he already knows that somehow this isn't ideal. He has to be quick as Andrea is always waiting for him and isn't supposed to know about his detour to the restroom.

"Usually," I say, "a tense orgasm means less pleasure. Is that so in your case?"

"I do enjoy it, but mainly because of the relaxation afterward. But otherwise, it really is difficult to . . . come." He grins sheepishly.

Harold also tells me how when he's masturbating, he braces his legs against the wall opposite his seat, really pressing, holding his breath and rubbing quickly. And all this with as little noise as possible, meaning mute button on—not only the iPad, but also on any of the moans he might let out.

Answering my question about muscular tension, he says his upper body and neck are strained; his position while masturbating reminds him of a bow. While all this is happening, the dog waits outside the door: he can't let it into the house first as his wife would wonder what happened to him.

Even though his story has a funny side, even the slightest smile on my part would be inappropriate. Blame and shame are written all over Harold's face. He looks as though he feels like a swine, an unfaithful coward, which he immediately confirms when I raise the topic.

When he later describes the situation that led to the first appointment with me, his mood brightens a bit. One evening after his wife went to bed, she got up again to make herself a cup of tea. She suddenly thought she heard the dog. She called her: "Tussiiiie!" That's the name the children chose for their pretty golden-brown collie with a bushy lion-like mane and white "socks." "Tussiiiie!"

And what else would you expect? Tussie barked back from the outbuilding. The master was discovered, caught in the act. Pants down around the ankles, he staggered out of the unlocked restroom, the iPad still glowing on the counter. It showed two young ladies dressed in sexy underwear, licking and kissing each other while enticingly looking in the eyes of the viewer—in this case, now, Andrea, who from then on has considered Harold to be perverted.

Harold stood there broken, his wife looking at him in disbelief with tears in her eyes.

"Well, at least she didn't catch me with my hand in my pants." He smiles at me shyly, and even I can't disguise my amusement.

"And I used to think of the Lassie movies as romantic," I say. "Dog saves man."

He understands what I meant straight away.

"Have you talked it over?" I ask, serious again.

"No. Andrea just said that she'd been worried about me, that I'd been away for so long. And that was all. In bed she turned away from me, although we always snuggle together." He continues: "Since then, every evening after I've done the round with the dog, I see it in her face."

"What do you see?"

"How she's suffering from thinking about what I've done in the bathroom . . ."

"Are you sure? Have you ever asked her?"

"No..."

"I would very much like to ask your wife about it when the three of us are here. Maybe she'll mention it during her solo appointment. May I use your version of the story freely?"

"You can tell her everything I've said—after all, we *have* decided to take this path." Harold seems relieved.

The next thing I want to know from him is whether he's masturbated at all since then. He answers that he has, but only once a week, when Andrea is at her yoga class and the children are in bed—still after taking the dog for a walk and in the aforementioned restroom.

In the course of the session it becomes increasingly clear from Harold's descriptions where his still great problem maintaining an erection originated. He noticed that when he's watching porn, he's only interested in faces. "The women have to look nice and be pretty. I don't look down below." He's got used to this form of arousal. He also says that when it comes sex, it's no longer primarily about actual intercourse for him but that he would prefer to stroke his wife's clitoris or satisfy her orally. (In both cases there's no need for an erection!)

"That's just the problem," he says. "Even then she doesn't have an orgasm. Her coming when being stroked is important to me." It's plain that Harold feels like a failure. He's been trying very hard to sexually arouse his wife, and along the way he has forgotten his penis, which in any case has not really been cooperating.

"Your wife hasn't learned to come yet." I consciously choose a formulation in which the responsibility rests on Andrea. Harold grudgingly agrees. Then I say, "I would like to see you again alone so that we can talk about techniques for improving your arousal."

Harold seems lost in his thoughts, then: "I have a guilty conscience because Andrea hasn't felt my penis inside her for such a long time. She used to like it a lot."

I promise him that we will cover all these topics and end the session.

As we're saying our goodbyes, I say, "I would certainly call the next dog Lassie."

He grins and hits the road.

Afterward I think about how things were between Harold and Andrea. Harold literally let his pants down. Both were ashamed; neither spoke about it. But both Harold and Andrea can read faces.

Going Down

"HOW ARE YOU?" I ask as Andrea arrives for her individual session. In contrast to Harold, she is here on the dot. This time she's wearing a longer denim skirt with a soft, draping blouse, her dark hair tied in a ponytail—a pretty, hippie-chic look.

"Good!" she says. "The last session was very interesting."

"Why?"

"Hmm . . . I really didn't realize how much we were holding stuff back. And then speaking about it wasn't bad at all. Just the opposite."

"After the appointment did you talk more at home?"

"No, but the atmosphere has changed since then."

"That's nice." I then want to talk to Andrea about her sexuality, and decide to approach the sensitive subject directly.

"Your husband has an iPad, doesn't he?"

"Oh, has he told you *that* story?" Andrea has mapped me well.

"Yes, and he said that I could talk it over with you." With this information I want to show her that I remain professionally discrete. There's no way she should get the impression that I'm bonding with her behind her husband's back.

"He feels very bad about what he did," she explains, which gives me cause to believe that she isn't going to like my answer to her comment, namely, that her husband—in my opinion—can masturbate when, where, and for whatever reason he likes. At least it would be good if he could, and here I think things have to be put straight.

"Your husband thinks you didn't approve of his toilet escapade," I say.

"Right. I thought it was disgusting."

"What don't you like about it?"

"I have a problem with the fact that my partner does it alone."

"That's not the first time I've heard that. Why is it that way with you?"

"If he feels sexually aroused, then he should do it with *me*. Otherwise, I feel like I'm not enough for him."

"Maybe you're right. Maybe you really *aren't* enough for him."

"Is that possible?" She looks shocked.

"Of course! But would that be too bad?"

She describes her views about what marriage partners should do for each other and with each other.

"It seems," I say, "as though your husband manages to look after himself pretty well. That's great, isn't it?"

"Errr, well, maybe it is . . . Probably."

She seems unsure, so we stay on the subject. We talk about how each person can do as they please, can enjoy sex alone, and I get the impression that slowly she begins reconsidering her thoughts. Slowly.

"But does he have to watch porn, of all things?" She looks as if even she finds the question a bit odd, at the very least. Then she puts it another way: "Doesn't he want *me* anymore?"

"Under certain circumstances, you could say that, but do you ever feel that he *doesn't* want to have sex with you?"

"Oh no! Not at all. From the very beginning Harold has wanted more sex than me. I often feel better—without sex," she says, adding meekly, "Maybe he's just annoyed with me because of the fuss I make."

"Do you touch yourself?" I ask in a friendly manner but still firmly.

"Oh God, no!"

"Nice of you to mention Him!"

"Who?"

"You know, the one who didn't have sex," I say grinning, "and had His son produced by the Holy Ghost."

"Did I say God?"

Then I get serious again. "Yes, and *He* really doesn't have anything to do with it." Spontaneously I decide to change tack. "Or maybe He does. Are you ashamed?"

She nods. "I think sex is part of marriage—well, that's what I learned, anyway—and if all alone he—"

I interrupt Andrea: "So, your husband should act on his sexual desires with you?" She nods. "But you don't usually have any." And here I end my objection.

There is almost a minute of silence. Neither of us says anything. I can literally feel how Andrea's deeply entrenched notions of sex and marriage begin to crumble.

"Basically," she says, "it suits us pretty well. Even though it's a bit sad."

I back her up. "Yes, and it's not necessary to wear a moral corset. Shame can also be a clamp imposed by society." I smile. "So that we don't all spend our time screwing around."

My statement hasn't seemed to have convince her (yet), so she tries another argument.

"Sex is an extremely emotional thing, and a person shouldn't treat it lightly. Of course, it can be fun, but you also have to set limits and not to take things too far. For me, sex is part of a relationship."

"Okay, but in every relationship there are two partners, and they don't always have the same opinions and needs. Which needs are *you* satisfying when you're having sex?"

As if it was self-evident, she answers, "The need to let feelings run free, to gain trust and love, to have a sense of belonging and oneness."

It sounds like a shopping list.

They're all emotional needs linked to love, all stored "upstairs." I ask Andrea whether she can imagine speaking about genital needs. She remained "upstairs." She talked about her own sexuality, her cravings, and above all her inhibitions.

"What do you associate with your 'down below'?" I usually use the word *vulva* for female genitalia, but if I chose that word with Andrea at this stage, it's conceivable that I wouldn't reach her. I consider it better to borrow her terminology, which, in due course, I can guide in a more sensual direction.

"I think society nowadays is far too superficial. Everyone's too easygoing, only interested in the physical side of things. I miss the spiritual side." And suddenly we're "upstairs" again.

I try again. "I want to go *doooown!*"

Andrea answers promptly: "A lot of people brush feelings and emotions aside, just live for the day. This is wrong as far as I'm concerned. Maybe that's why I'm a bit strict about sex."

"Are you not also brushing something aside?"

"I don't think so . . ."

"I've been trying to steer your attention downward, and it seems to me that you're avoiding this at all costs."

"It's possible," she admits.

"Down below is very important for arousal and lust," I explain. "Lust does indeed begin in the head, but we *feel* it down below. Some women, however, are said to still believe that it's dirty, or even forbidden."

During my explanation I observe once again how difficult it is for Andrea to cast her eyes "south." But evidently, I've managed to gradually win her over, as all of a sudden she says, "I think sperm is disgusting, and actually, the penis too." She contorts her face—even the thought of them seems to trigger revulsion. I remember that Harold said in his individual session that when she masturbates him, her upper body moves ever farther away and her arm gets longer and longer. After he comes, she wipes her wet hand on him and then goes immediately to the restroom to wash herself off.

Again I reassure Andrea, telling her that this feeling is common among women, that not everyone associates their partners' organs with sexual desire. But they can learn to. And for their part, many men are not particularly concerned with the delights of the vulva or vagina.

I try to discover what Andrea thinks about her vulva or vagina, whether she knows them well, and it turns out that she has never explored or touched herself there (she

68

links this to revulsion too). After showering, Andrea always dresses quickly without looking in the mirror. She doesn't want to look at herself. Sex with Harold always takes place in the dark.

This is, unfortunately, not uncommon. Astonishingly, many women have never really been interested in their sexual organs, haven't even properly looked there.

"Well," I say, "what *does* your vulva look like? Would you recognize it in the Lost and Found?"

For her homework, we agree that she should take a good look "down below," almost as if she's going to make a detailed drawing. Also, every morning before getting up and every evening before going to sleep, she should lovingly place her hand on her vulva and say "good morning" or "good night" to the "new" part of her body. And finally I tell her about a colleague named Ella Berlin. Ella wanted her four daughters to find a name for their genitalia—and it had to be a good one. She knew about the Sanskrit word *yoni* from tantric sex practices, but she was looking for a word without esoteric connotations. She considered the term for the external female organ—*vulva*—and then for the internal one—the *vagina*. Without further ado, she combined the two and the word *vulvina* was born—a beautiful birth!

5

The Best in Us, the Worst in Us

K RISTEN WAS ROUGHLY FIFTY, and in her younger days could have been a model. Now she had heavily made-up eyes and a figure somewhere between slender and ample. Her husband, Michael, was twenty years older, but I never got to meet him, as Kristen always came alone to my office. Michael was a rich and successful businessman—he had really made it. He was still very much involved with his company: although he was past retirement age, he had little time to share with Kristen. Their three children, brought up over the years almost solely by Kristen, were grown up and had long moved away from home.

Sometimes in their large—and now in many ways empty—house, unpleasant things happened. Kristen told me that during a dinner party with friends, for instance, Michael abruptly cut her short: "Darling, I'm still the one who pays for our lifestyle, so could you just shut up?" Which Kristen proceeded to do, because if it came to divorce, she would be almost penniless—a prenuptial agreement had taken care of that. On the one hand, she was financially dependent on him, but on the other, she couldn't really claim that she was suffering with her life of luxury. Her expensive clothes, sporty coupe, beautiful trips abroad, healthy credit card . . . Michael granted her all that. But among friends or in the little time that they were alone together, he was always nagging her. For instance, her new handbag: it must have swallowed a whole month's wages!

When Kristen described her husband, it wasn't only that he subtly criticized his wife. His taunts were so explicit that even with the best will in the world, it was impossible to ignore them. Michael seemed to be a real brute.

Mutual sex was also a thing of the past. Michael wanted nothing more to do with "emotional things"—they just distracted from other, more important things. For Kristen it seemed as though Michael had decided that they would never sleep together again, just like that. Did he not want to, or couldn't he? Was he trying to punish her? Whatever the case, there didn't seem to be any signs of sexual interest on his part, although she went to a lot of trouble to make herself look good for him, in the hope that he would notice it.

"In the meantime, everything is too much of an effort for him," she said while giving me the impression that she was just about to join him there. On the few occasions that she had fought against Michael's rejection, such as by trying to hug him, he brushed her off with a swish of the hand as if shooing away an annoying fly, causing her to remark, "You're getting old, Michael."

"You too, Kristen," was his response.

Kristen was deeply frustrated and unhappy but didn't have the strength or courage to separate or to talk things over with her husband. For financial reasons, for convenience, because of the children—always the same excuses. If Kristen was really in tune with her feelings and wishes, she could no longer have remained passive.

One thing she definitely wasn't in favor of: totally waiving sex. She still felt far too young for that. She and Michael had long slept in separate rooms, but every now and then they used to visit each other and spend the night together. At some stage, however, even this small diversion had ended.

Kristen could shop or meet up with friends as much as she liked, but that wasn't a substitute for sex. Her days were unfulfilled. She considered her position. Okay, her husband didn't feel like having sex, but she could have a lover, some adventure or other that would brighten up her gloomy housewife routine (of course, they had household staff).

Kristen began a few fleeting affairs, which always ended before things were allowed to get too serious—she was well aware that as far as her husband was concerned, she wasn't showing herself in the best light. Initially she very much enjoyed the affection and physical release with her mostly younger lovers. She felt wanted, alive, and appreciated, all the things that she had recently been missing with Michael.

Gradually, however, she became troubled by a guilty conscience, and didn't know what she should do. Basically, she still wanted sex with her husband and the father of their children.

"But I still love Michael!"

I asked her what love meant to her: "Something to be inspired by? Being well treated, or badly treated? Being prosperous? Being humiliated in front of friends?"

Her answer: "Sometimes he can be really nice..."

Kristen had obviously never really thought hard about what love meant to her. Her words seemed to be an escape. A simple declaration of love would never have crossed her lips—she wouldn't have allowed it. She also didn't have to tell me: I could see it in how she looked at her bag on the sofa (it really was a stunning handbag, but you can buy some perfectly good cloth bags), the pictures on the wall, her glass of water on the table... She managed to skillfully avoid my eyes.

Your Partner's Choice

I COULD ONLY give her one piece of advice: "At some stage you're going to have to be honest with your husband—or remain silent. But you have to be able to live with your choice." After a short pause I continued: "You've begun to lie. One day your husband will get wind of it and he's unlikely to be happy about it."

"You're quite right." Kristen looked miserable. "But he kept putting me down."

"The world is often unfair, but that's no reason for you to remain silent. You've never clearly let your husband know that you don't want to be treated like that. Respect is important in a relationship, seeing eye to eye."

When partners finally talk about themselves and their relationship honestly and, unlike before, have something serious to say, the other person notices the difference. It no longer matters that earlier reactions were dismissive, that there were threats of divorce or of acting on a premarital contract. There's no going back; things have started to roll, and something has happened that each side knows fundamentally involves them both.

I had to confront Kristen with another possible reaction from Michael: "Have you ever considered that your husband might look for a younger replacement?"

Kristen opened her eyes wide in horror at the thought, although, as she said, the question wasn't new for her.

Of course, I could have presented my views differently, with a little more padding or some filler. I could have also reacted with more empathy, a little more understanding of her lifestyle, I could have encouraged her when she was describing Michael to me by agreeing that he really was a blockhead. But behavior that appears to be soothing and understanding on my part wouldn't have helped Kristen recognize her living situation for what it was—unacceptable.

Whatever Kristen chose to do, she didn't return for therapy. But she did thank me by email for my clear words and honesty. Time and again I think of her and the handbag that she ostentatiously placed on the sofa next to her as if saying, "Look at me!" But not in the way she intended—that she had a husband who was able to buy her such an exclusive handbag. No. Rather, she had a substitute husband, and this "handbag husband" was accompanying her to therapy in place of Michael.

All this reminds me of another client, a woman in her mid-forties whose story was similar. But she took things further. She told me that sometimes when she returned home late at night slightly tipsy, she had a "quickie at the front door" with her lover before climbing into bed with her husband. She arranged it all by phoning her lover from the cab on the way home. Despite her blunt language, she looked as if she felt ashamed, but apparently not enough to stop doing it.

"I simply summon my lover, who then comes for a quick screw." (She didn't pay him anything for his services.)

I got to the heart of the matter. "You screw while your husband is asleep upstairs—and you feel bad about it?"

"Yes, very."

"How would you describe a woman who does things like that if it wasn't you?"

"A slut?"

"That'd be one reasonable possibility."

Now, I'm not a moral arbiter—I don't wag my finger. I don't condemn affairs, be they in janitors' closets or fancy hotel rooms. Everyone can live out their passions and desires as often or as torridly as they wish. It's clear to me, though, that every secret affair has a certain aftertaste. The betrayed partner is cheated of choice, at least if monogamy was agreed upon—out loud or not. Keeping affairs secret is mostly a continuation of what was practiced throughout the time of living together: an inability to speak with one another. Think about it for a second. Would you be able to keep respecting your partner if they were casually cheating on you? And what if they've realized it but are too scared to do something about it? Or it simply wasn't important enough to mention? Secret flings undermine respect that in a relationship should *always* be there for both parties.

I constantly make sure that clients also keep their bad sides visible, the things that they don't want to see—*their* contribution to a problem, *their* share of responsibility that they are unwilling to accept. To do this I have to be prepared to provoke them or raise unpleasant truths, as our bad side rarely solves any problems for us. But being able to talk about our bad side is definitely a strength: only the best in us can identify the worst in us; the worst in us will even deny its own existence.

It's not a matter of what the neighbors could be whispering or what others think of you, but rather that even when you're brushing your teeth, you can look yourself in the eye. That you're comfortable with yourself, true to yourself. Time and again it makes me think . . . how often people neglect their fear of being abandoned. Crazy! The Devil with his devilish plan—you can't say that it didn't succeed. He must be really proud of his PR machinery.

The Language of Emotions

LIFE, LIKE THERAPY, is all about being aware of needs and feelings. And although for many people these don't have anything to do directly with sex, they're still part of the picture, because when we're aware of our feelings and learn to understand them, we're better able to look after them and are better prepared to take on more responsibility. And this also applies to sex. There are a few basic emotions, positive and negative: joy, anger, sadness, disgust, fear, shame, contempt, and surprise. Are clients even able to identify these emotions in themselves? Whereabouts in the body do they feel them? Is it possible to withstand an emotion? Clients often think that they can talk about a situation with their partner only after they completely understand it. But who ever does?

What about this: Everyone knows how it feels when something isn't right. Maybe you're suddenly sad or angry; you would prefer to distance yourself a bit. A couple can arrange things so that that when feelings like this arise in one of them, there is a certain reaction—regardless of whether what's behind those feeling is clear or not. "I became a bit sad just as you said that!" Afterward the couple can think about how to continue. Do we want to talk? Or should we wait? Or—in the positive sense—was that it? It's often enough just to mention something for that thing to be straightened out. In any case, it's good that both know what the mood is.

I try to make clients conscious about which needs or feelings they are neglecting. I show them how it's possible to improve contact with each other, and also how intimate moments can develop if they show their vulnerability. It is exactly this intimacy that many people fear.

We aren't used to carefully appreciating our emotions. But emotions, even bad ones, are trying to tell us something. Feelings are treasures! Feelings are expecting us to react. Do it!

6

Whiteout:

BLURRED
BOUNDARIES

SOMETIMES, ALTHOUGH NOT often, I don't manage to find a new way for a client. Not because they decide to cut therapy short—that would be a conscious decision I can and have to accept.

No—sometimes I can't seem to bring light to darkness with my tools, such as when a client is suffering from what I call "whiteout."

In the polar regions there is a meteorological phenomenon in which outlines and contours become indistinct in the surrounding mist, snow, and diffuse sunlight. The horizon disappears; there are no shadows; sky and ground form a seamless entity; everything is without boundaries. This is called "whiteout," and those who have experienced it know how threatening it can be as there's a serious risk of totally losing orientation and getting lost or injured in endless icefields. The safest approach for avoiding danger is to wait exactly where you are in the hope that the situation will improve.

A similar phenomenon is known in neuropsychology. Sufferers fail to recognize an established reality and in its place a blind spot appears. Take, for example, Shayne.

Shayne was roughly forty, a powerfully built man with a slightly angular face, short, stubbly hair, and a job as a paramedic. He could have looked self-confident had he not had an expression so dejected that it transformed his appearance to the very opposite. The father of two had not come to the practice of his own free will. His wife of eleven years, Marie, had asked him to visit me, and he had obeyed her instructions. She thought something wasn't quite right with her husband.

"Did your wife describe it in a little more detail?" I inquired.

"She said it pretty clearly." Shayne lowered his head. "She wants me to seduce her and do something about my limp erection. Apart from that, we don't speak to each other much." He looked up again.

My new client gave me the impression that he didn't mind that at all, the not speaking to each other—nothing unusual, unfortunately.

Shayne told me that he was once an alcoholic but that he had been dry for many years. Additionally, I heard that privately, things weren't going too well: his wife had started having an affair with a colleague—at the company Shayne too worked at—five months earlier. But he wasn't here because of that.

"Do you and your wife still have sex with each other?"

"Not for a long time, partly because I just don't feel like it. My wife used to stimulate me, but that's gone down the last three or four years. She tells me she wants me to be more active. She wants more sex where *I'm* the initiator. And more talking."

"And she didn't say anything more?"

"No. But she's right, isn't she?"

His wife was concerned about both the quality and the quantity of sex, and she'd clearly got her point across. I suspected, however, that her real purpose was to provoke a reaction from her husband, to finally wake him up.

I didn't follow up on his question. Instead I wanted to hear from him how he'd come to know that his wife was having an affair.

"Through her itemized cellphone bill. I opened the envelope by mistake because I use the same provider. I asked Marie why she called a certain number so often, whether she had someone else. She admitted right away that she had been having an affair with a coworker."

"Did she then say that she would end it?"

"No, she didn't. She asked for time to think things over, to think about how to carry on."

So, Shayne's wife needed time. Actually, I thought to myself, coping with situations like this is always difficult. You have to wait even though you don't want to do so. The uncertainty eats away at you. However, it was a good sign that Marie didn't try to deny it all. She could have claimed that she and the associate were completing an important project and that the phone calls were part of that. The fact that she was up front about the affair told me that she needed a change and was now prepared to take her chances.

"How important is your family to you?" I asked her husband.

"Very important. It's just that at the moment I have the feeling that every step that I make is like dancing on a razor's edge."

Razor's edge, a phrase conjuring up many images, few of them good. And at the same time, his wife was dancing on clouds, hovering above a volcano that was ready to erupt at any moment.

"So your wife is still sleeping with her colleague?"

"I don't know. She hides her cellphone from me." He spoke almost in a whisper. By the way, if you are thinking right now that Shayne's wife was *still* having an affair, you probably successfully mapped not only Shayne but also his wife. How can I be so sure? Because I just mind mapped *you* reading these lines!

Shayne came to me for almost two years, at irregular intervals. His wife, who had originally sent him to me, didn't come even once, and also wasn't interested in what we talked about in the sessions. She continued to show not the slightest interest in his feelings. The situation put a strain on him. He had deep, dark rings beneath his eyes, and appeared tired and listless. But he wasn't tired because he'd been digging up his garden or chopping down trees—he was tired because of the emotional burden. His wife couldn't have missed it but still didn't offer any support or reveal her progress on her "time to think things over" regarding their relationship. I began to form an impression of Marie, and it wasn't a pleasant one—rather one of a brutal and very egotistical woman.

Time and again Shayne was overcome by great sorrow while telling his story. He would sit there head bowed, breathing heavily, as if he was having to drag himself through life. He looked like a maltreated dog that had been beaten so often that it had lost the will to fight back.

As I raised the subject of his posture, Shayne said that his coworkers had already been asking him if he was ill. He always waved them off—how was he supposed to explain to them what was really going on? Even in my office, talking about himself and his situation was agonizing. He was unable to pose the liberating question that he wanted to ask his wife: "Is your affair still on?" He was too afraid of the answer, which could have been: "Yes, and that's why I want a divorce." Living with Marie in this unbearable situation was preferable to risking the truth. All he had to do was look at the shift schedule to know when his wife would be continuing the affair. *Sex by the shift schedule* passed through my mind. It was also how Shayne and his wife had come to know each other. For me, Shayne was a man sitting in a burning house. He preferred to roast alive inside his four trusty walls rather than run through the flames to freedom. With her breach of faith, Marie had presented him with a fait accompli, and he was simply unable to face his remaining options. He sat there, firmly trapped in the dilemma.

Nothing changed, not even in the ensuing months. Marie and Shayne continued not having sex and not talking to each other. On the other hand, Marie *was* having sex and *was* speaking to someone—it just wasn't Shayne.

"Let's talk about the time before the affair started," I said eventually. "Were you really not lacking anything then?"

"Marie said I was lacking manliness."

That wasn't what I'd meant with that question! I had to grin.

"What do you think of as 'manliness'?"

"Not hiding your light under a bushel."

This expression was probably taken word for word from Marie. I've heard it many times from women who wish their men didn't give up so easily or that they stood by an opinion. "Softies" like Shayne, however, find all that somehow macho and reject it outright for themselves. Shayne also felt awkward when he held a different opinion from his wife. Marie could get very angry, he said. He was afraid of any unpleasantness and, ultimately, afraid of losing her.

Gradually I tried to make it plain that he had to take the plunge and talk about unpleasant matters. He had to start talking with his wife, to offer to be a real counterpart to her in the relationship. He nodded and remembered something that Marie had once said to him: "It's as if you're not even here. I can do whatever I want—you never say anything." Exactly. In the end she could pretty much do whatever she wanted and he still wouldn't say anything. He had become resigned to her impositions even though he was suffering miserably. Marie was putting Shayne to the test, and in selecting a lover she had posed the hardest question. She wanted to know where she stood with her husband. There were more gentle ways to do this, but she had decided on this one. She probably didn't have much left to lose.

I was certain that Shayne had blown the test. He had set her no limits when the affair was confirmed. She must have expected anger, accusations, pain—but they failed to materialize. Shayne, like a tortoise, had retreated into his shell. Marie's feeling had been confirmed—she lived side by side with a nobody who wasn't interested in what she did.

Of course, that wasn't so—things were festering, his sorrow and fears were eating away at him. He felt remote controlled, and was worried that one day the sex that Marie was having with their colleague would turn to love. Without thinking, he continued monitoring Marie's phone bills when he could in the hope that the number of calls and messages would decrease. There was only one consolation, and a small one at that: the man his wife was seeing wasn't unattached—he too was married with children.

In the meantime, Shayne was "reading" his wife almost obsessively, looking for signs that Marie had ended the affair. Although he could hardly bear the strain, he still hadn't confronted her. It was enough for him when from time to time she casually touched him—in the kitchen before dinner, or while they decorated the Christmas tree for the kids, or wrapped birthday presents. One evening they even watched a rom-com on TV together holding hands. Sometimes he gave her a playful slap on her bum. She was okay with that. More, he couldn't say.

In therapy Shayne practiced confronting his wife, by role playing. Sometimes I took on Marie's role, sometimes his. I always felt that these role-playing sessions were helpful for him. After one session he even wrote his wife a letter, but he never gave it to her.

He was still simply unable to take the bull by the horns. What was blocking this man? Why couldn't he go on the offensive? Time and again I felt that the therapy wasn't focused enough. However, he assured me that the talks with me were helping; every time he felt slightly better, although this is not always a good sign.

And so he slowly progressed with my assistance, from Easter to Labor Day, from birthdays to Christmas to Valentine's Day. He kept the anger, which he must have had, under lock and key like Her Majesty's crown jewels.

Apropos crown jewels—one detail particularly bothered me. Shayne hadn't even considered abandoning the marriage bed. He continued sleeping next to Marie, the one who was being unfaithful. Not only that: he did it naked.

"I think your behavior is a bit odd," I said to him when he told me this.

He looked at me astonished. "What's so strange about it?"

"Well," I answered, "you're showing Marie your penis, in which she's no longer interested because she has another man's . . . She has someone else's penis." Once again I tried to increase the pressure, tried to force Shayne out of this stalemate.

"Well, what's wrong about that?"

"There's nothing wróng about it, but doesn't it bother you that every evening your crown jewels are dangling in front of the very woman who wants nothing to do with them?" Shayne obviously was hardly aware that his penis, as a sexual object, was actually a part of him. I restated my position: "I wouldn't like my partner parading such intimate parts of himself in front of me if we were no longer sexually attracted."

Slowly glimmers of light appeared. "You think I should put something on before I go to bed?"

So the ball was back in my court. Instead of finding the answer for himself and standing by it, Shayne was hoping for my advice. I returned the ball by saying he should make up his own mind.

Shayne looked at me, head inclined. "I should put something on before getting into bed?" he repeated cautiously.

He read me correctly, and once again I had unintentionally made his decision.

I wondered—and not for the first time—whether it would have been different if we had worked on Shayne's sexual "staying power" and the feeling of masculinity linked to this. Doing so often leads to the client taking more responsibility for his own actions, even outside of the bedroom, and in multiple ways achieving some sort of standing. But Shayne had flatly refused to have anything to do with this form of physical therapy—right from the very beginning. His erectile dysfunction remained unspoken; his only topic of discussion was and remained his wife's affair. I, however, persisted in my questions.

It became increasingly clear that there must be something specific behind his self-destructive behavior, something that probably went way back. I had discovered that Shayne's parents were alcoholics—it was no accident that he too had been drinking a lot. He had also explained that his mother was mentally unstable. Sometimes she was prepared to pick fights; other times she was depressed and just loafed around lethargically. In this state she often reacted harshly and disproportionately. She used to be like this often. When Shayne was young he learned to leave his mother be and to withdraw into silence. At least then he felt that his own little world remained intact even when everything around him was threatening to collapse.

Shayne's shield against his family explained a number of things: it was his way of dealing with problems. He used the same strategy with his wife. But for me it was still puzzling that he wasn't able to shift his perspective, to take another stance, in order to recognize how much he was suffering from his situation and maybe to seek relief from it. What was crippling him?

Shayne was convinced that he was going in the right direction, that there had been slight improvements. He told me that recently Marie had left her phone lying around. The number of text messages had dropped. The fact that he referred to this development as hugely positive meant to me that Shayne was still interested in only one thing: continuing to deceive himself into believing that his difficult marriage still existed—no matter how dysfunctional it was. If Marie didn't want sex with him, that was perfectly okay, as long as she stayed with him. Eventually Shayne began to seriously tell me that he was now quite satisfied with the situation...but he continued to make appointments with me. This couple never ceased to astonish me. By getting her sex elsewhere, Marie was doing exactly the same thing as Shayne: steering well clear of their actual problem, their mutual relationship. But it wasn't only Marie who was ignoring Shayne—he was ignoring himself. I decided that things couldn't carry on like this.

At the very next session I told Shayne that we could continue to work together only if he did what had to be done: confront Marie about the affair—assuming Marie really meant something to him, which he roundly confirmed.

"Come back when you've taken this step—by all means, with Marie."

Shayne was silent for a long time. Then he began to talk, very quietly, while looking at me almost pleadingly, as if he was expecting encouragement. I nodded at him—I definitely didn't want him to stop talking.

"At fifteen, maybe sixteen, I wanted to go out one night with a couple of buddies. Some girls were supposed to be joining us. I was wearing a new T-shirt and a cool jacket. I was in the hall when I saw my mother at the top of the staircase." Shayne faltered, seeking the right words. "I went to the stairs to say goodbye."

"And what happened next?" I asked.

"She walked down the stairs and planted herself in front of me on the bottom stair so we were the same height. But it wasn't like it was usually—it felt really strange. She said, 'I see you're going out. Have you ever kissed anyone properly?' I said no, was absolutely terrified that my mother had asked a question like that. Before I understood what was happening, she said, 'I'll show you.' Then she grabbed my head in both hands and kissed me . . . long and with her tongue. I didn't resist, just let it happen. It was totally disgusting."

Shayne was quiet, breathing with difficulty, gazing at the floor with his hands knotted. I could see what a huge inward struggle he was having. I was sure that at that time, despite his physical advantage, he had no chance of avoiding his mother. Emotionally she had him completely under her control. Because of this I asked him the next question.

"Do you think you could have avoided her advances?"

"I was way too shocked."

"I can well believe that."

And from that moment, I was sure that I knew Shayne's problem. He was suffering from whiteout. At the moment of traumatization the victim can think, but cognitive functions slow and short-term memory breaks down. The person feels as if they're in a tunnel or a thick fog: whiteout. Shayne's mind mapping collapsed with every horrifying situation in which he was unable to defend himself against his mother's sexual abuse. His brain suffered whiteout—like Superman with kryptonite.

He was unable to come to terms with the fact that his own mother was able to inflict such harm and disgust—and intentionally. She knew exactly what she was doing, could put herself in his position. She had read him and went precisely for the spot that would cause the most damage.

Disgust is a primary emotion. This means that it is not acquired but is deeply anchored in the brain across cultures. It is an involuntary physical reaction that causes us to distance ourselves as quickly and as far from the source of disgust as possible. The trouble is, how is this possible when the source is your own mother? After all, you're dependent on her. So Shayne's mind-mapping system masked the truth that his mother was monstrous. Likewise, it masked the fact that he had been sickened and would preferred to have fled the scene as quickly as possible. It created a blind spot—and was most likely when the issue of relationships with women arose.

I was happy that Shayne had made an important step toward recovery. He had just proved to himself, within the protective bounds of therapy, that he was able to admit what had happened long ago on the stairs.

"It didn't do me much good at that time, did it," he said in a quiet voice.

"What are you thinking?" I asked. He didn't answer. "Did you want the kiss?"

"No, it was revolting."

"Could you have done anything against it?"

"I didn't have the slightest chance."

"That's right."

Shayne couldn't have avoided his mother at that time. And the traumatized link to her had plagued him all his life. His subsequent relationships were seriously affected by it. During the seemingly endless seconds that his mother had kissed him against his will, he had made a defining experience that people he trusted could hurt him and even get pleasure or satisfaction from it. From then on this applied not only to his relationships to his mother but to those with anyone close to him—including, or particularly, his wife. Did she not do precisely what his mother did? She tormented Shayne, and deliberately. And just as in his earlier trauma on the staircase, he chose to stand without defense in whiteout rather take a rash step toward the abyss.

Blind spots have their price. They hamper people, particularly when it comes to their development. Shayne was able to understand some things but not others—not how horribly his wife treated him, for instance. Had he been able to, he probably would have recognized that they had to separate or renegotiate their relationship dynamics. But he couldn't. When women went beyond Shayne's boundaries, he didn't accuse them. Just the opposite: he defended them.

He said his mother had an unhappy childhood. That could well have been true, but it still didn't justify what she'd done.

After that session Shayne didn't contact me again, and I wasn't expecting him to. He had reached a slightly higher step in his consciousness and now saw the situation with Marie for what it was, and his fear of the next necessary step—talking to his wife—was all the greater. At this point, at least, he was satisfied with what he had achieved: Marie was still with him.

Maybe you're thinking that it was best not to continue with Shayne, as he could have become depressed if he carried on grappling with everything he had been through. But this is not necessarily true. If the right form of therapy is chosen, if the patient is neither over-extended nor under-extended, change can happen more quickly and more profoundly than most people expect. Humans are robust; humans are resilient. As a therapist, these are forces that I address.

7

When to Go, When to Stay

MANY YEARS AGO a relationship of mine was about to end: breakup was imminent. I was going way beyond my limits with my boyfriend at that time, Peter; friends and family were worried about me, I was losing weight and looking bad. But still I considered it worthwhile not to give up completely—there was still hope. At least Peter and I were looking for a solution to our problems and were talking to each other.

At the beginning of our relationship we had been very symbiotic, always together, pleasing and endorsing each other the whole day long. Putting it positively, we were in love, and helping to bring out the best in each other. But even then, right from the start, there were warning signs. Peter often felt hurt and offended. Apparently I often wounded his feelings without realizing how and when. Then he would go into a sulk lasting days on end. What, with hindsight, we should have learned from each other was that Peter should have had more clearly defined limits and I should have accepted them. We tried talking about it, but appearances are deceptive: Peter, after a three-year relationship, had already inwardly distanced himself, which he denied when challenged. He was so scared of splitting up that he couldn't talk about it. We were still in love. At the same time, Peter spurned not only sex but any form of affection that could have brought us together again. I wasn't even allowed to touch him anymore. And me? I was always letting him off the hook, telling myself that everything would be okay and that I just had to be patient. I was on the way to being blinded by love.

"Why don't we separate?" I asked him. "Given you don't want anything to do with me." He wasn't ready yet, was his reply. There was still love. Fifty-fifty. Even this half-love Peter was unable to live out with me. From time to time I was almost frantic about the different messages he was sending. On the one hand, he seemed to still like me a lot and wanted to stay in our relationship; on the other hand, he wanted nothing to do with what *makes* a relationship—no physical contact, no shared time, no closeness. The situation got worse; I didn't remain complacent but spoke with Peter over and over again about our impossible situation.

Then, with one single sentence from Peter, I was painfully conscious that it was a waste of time to continue hoping. At that time we had again become slightly closer, over the course of almost a month. Peter invited me to his place; we went to movies and concerts together; we were getting on just fine and even spent some nights together. We didn't have sex, however, and didn't kiss. Occasionally Peter commented about how nice it was to be together and, as he kept saying, how much he liked having me around. My hopes were beginning to grow. But then there was a situation in the kitchen.

Peter had invited me to his place for dinner. He was just about to grill a steak when I felt, by the way he was looking and moving, like he actually would have preferred to spend the evening without me—maybe even *because* we were beginning to get closer again. In retrospect it seems to me as if every time we began to get closer, he *had* to spurn me, as if he was frightened of getting lost or even vanishing in the relationship.

On this particular evening, when I reminded him that recently he had often noted how well we were getting on, Peter said, "I have no idea what you're talking about, Ann-Marlene. I've seen absolutely nothing good about us lately." The sentence wasn't said to provoke me or to start a quarrel, but was intended to simply be honest. I saw in Peter's face that he really meant it. He looked so cold, and it broke my heart. Our true feelings over the last few months had apparently been widely divergent. But when Peter couldn't even trust what *he* felt and said to me himself during our better moments, there was really nothing more I could do. I knew at that very second that there was no point in carrying on. The idea of "Peter and me" collapsed.

We separated affectionately and without having new lovers standing by. A simple "aha" moment, literally in the middle of a sentence, triggered the end—a private "aha" moment for me: now or never.

The pain was immense. I had to force myself to eat; I lost even more weight, shut myself indoors, and cried for months—every day a little less, but it was a long time. Since then I have known how real heartache feels. It was four years before I fell in love again, with my current partner. And Peter? I still love him—as much as it's possible to love someone you're no longer with. He is still part of my life.

In the last six months of my difficult relationship with Peter, I read a book by the American couples and sex therapist David Schnarch, *Intimacy & Desire,* in which he describes how to escape from symbiosis. It helped me before we split up and during the split. I remained true to myself and ended something that hadn't been doing me any good for a long time, although I knew how painful the end would be. The relationship itself and the crisis in it helped me to become more self-reliant, independent, and grown-up.

Schnarch calls the process I was going through during our breakup *differentiation.* Differentiation is measured on a scale that assesses a person's ability to balance out feelings and rationality, attachment (and intimacy) as well as autonomy in a relationship. One of the preconditions of differentiation is that each partner has a stable feeling of self-worth (not to be confused with self-confidence) that, despite intense physical and emotional closeness with the other person, remains intact. Should there be tensions in a relationship, those shouldn't lead to a loss in a partner's self-worth but rather should be endured, for as long as it makes sense to keep on trying. I had eventually arrived at the point where it didn't.

Schnarch identifies four aspects of differentiation:

1. SOLID, FLEXIBLE SELF
    You should be well aware of who you really are. This means asking yourself, *What do I want? What are my aims?* Depending on values and expectations, the

answers to this determine the actions you hold to be important and correct. Integrity also plays a role in the process. Someone can try to mess with me as much as they like—tug at me, goad me—but they won't have a chance: I won't let myself bend. I showed Peter that I wasn't willing to continue having a relationship that involved him distancing himself from me. This was the only way I could remain true to myself. A person with a solid self needs no external recognition for acceptance. The more solid a person's self-perception, the more explicitly they can show the way they are and what they want and need. Self-disclosure, being open about mistakes or weaknesses with a partner, belongs here too. I finally showed Peter how wounded and sad I was, but up to then I had mostly just been angry at him.

2. QUIET MIND, CALM HEART

In life, as in relationships, we need to be able to regulate our own fears and unpleasant feelings, and when stress does suddenly appear, we need to be able to remain calm. (Ha! That's quite a challenge for me.) The ability to be calm and console yourself, without outside help, in order to ease pain and control fear is particularly important. Then you aren't overwhelmed by your own emotional chaos. Life doesn't tear you apart. After our split, this was very important to me. I missed Peter bitterly, and every day I had to remind myself that at some point in the future, things were going to be all right—even if he was meeting other women and doing things with them that *I* wanted to do with him. I got to know a lot about what was going on and spent a lot of time thinking about myself and my life.

3. GROUNDED RESPONSE

When a relationship is going through a crisis, it can take a feat of strength not to overreact to the situation but to behave proportionally. This doesn't mean under-reacting or not reacting at all. Outside pressures and rejection have to be endured; those involved shouldn't explode or run away. Peter and I were far from such grounded emotional management. We were often in fight-or-flight mode, and had erected walls between us that were almost indestructible.

4. MEANINGFUL ENDURANCE

Crises have to be ridden out, no matter how painful disappointments, frustrations, and failures are for both partners. Setbacks should be conceded and then left behind; you have to be able to rise again and move on. Only then are you in the position to manage difficulties—and difficulties will inevitably arise. It's all about resilience, a strong and important human trait for developing good relationships, faith in yourself, and faith in others. Here too the opposite applies: you also need to do what has to be done when continuing no longer makes sense—as was the case for Peter and me.

Right and Important Endings

WITHOUT DIFFERENTIATION, WHICH I develop more and more and am teaching myself little by little, I wouldn't have separated from Peter then; we would probably have waited until we hated each other so much and caused each other so much pain that we wouldn't be able to get together today. I would have not really been myself for a much longer time and unable to keep an eye on my goals. I had to separate from Peter to survive. Afterward, I soothed my sorrows and licked my wounds without overreacting. At the same time, while very, very slowly getting over the pain of splitting up, I experienced everything consciously and with all my senses. This experience was an important step toward my future. This may sound odd, but it is not: yes, therapists, just like their clients, are human.

When I now see clients lying to themselves, it is my task to give them a good shake. I can do this because I know that I have experienced similar difficult feelings, and because I know what it feels like to see things clearly, even things that I don't like or want to see. My advice, and I seldom give advice, is be firm and weather it! Then you can stand erect—for your own good.

After Peter, I decided never to continue a love affair or relationship that no longer felt like one. People who remain in a relationship choose to continue feeling the way their relationship makes them feel. Mostly there is free will, and gradually there are choices to be made. Everyone is their own director. Nothing can be done just like that, as if by magic. Elizabeth and Chris should have discovered this the day they came to my practice.

The Night Owl and the Fitness Freak

ELIZABETH AND CHRIS came to my office together four times as well as booking individual sessions. Both were in their early to mid-thirties, and they had been a couple for seven years. Elizabeth was of medium height, somewhat shy in character with short dyed hair. She was slightly plump, which she concealed under an airy, colorful, patterned summer dress. She was a receptionist for a major TV station and mostly worked the night shift. Chris, a construction site manager, was in good shape, with muscles bulging beneath his shirt; he seemed to attach great importance to his body. He dressed sportily, in sneakers. His hands were sinewy, and his feet rocked on the floor as if he was about to start a hundred-meter race.

They had gotten to know each other on nights out, and at the beginning of their relationship they went out together many times. After they started their working lives, this lifestyle was possible only under exceptional circumstances. They had been sharing an apartment for two years. Their main problem, a common one: despite love, no sex. Elizabeth would have liked a little more intimacy; in this case, it was her partner who didn't feel like it. They had last slept together eight months earlier.

They had split up twice but each time got together again. The last split had been triggered by Elizabeth's continuing to lie about her alcohol consumption. Since then she had gone through therapy.

I was interested in hearing more about where the balance of desire between the two lay. To start with, I asked Chris, who wanted less sex than his partner.

Chris answered: "I don't feel much sexual desire, but I do have morning wood. And I masturbate at least three times a week."

He didn't actually sound like someone without sexual desires. The very opposite . . . Interesting.

Elizabeth said that she felt sexual desire. With sex she always had an orgasm, quickly and easily; she didn't have to exert herself. She had stopped taking the pill, and they had some problems with condoms because Chris's erection wasn't strong enough to slip them on.

Before I could continue with my questions, Chris said, "I used to think Elizabeth was sexy, but that's flagged. I'd like her to do something about her body."

Elizabeth looked away as he spoke—understandably, particularly as there was nothing wrong with her body. Of course, she wasn't as fit as her partner, somewhat softer and rounder, but a man like Chris could hardly be taken as a model for a woman. Their physical differences, however, didn't seem to be trouble-free for the two of them.

"When did sexual desire start to become difficult?"

Something had happened about two years earlier, around the time that they moved together—a fact that they both insisted had nothing to do with their problem. At that same time Chris had started to become interested in a new hobby—well, actually, a number of new ones. After Chris had started to feel that he would like to become a father and have children, he suddenly noticed how unhealthily they both lived and resolved to do something about it. Unfortunately, he somewhat overdid it. He started a number of different activities, like jogging, rock climbing, and swimming, all at once. On top of this, he went to the gym several times a week. He gave up smoking and changed his diet; not an ounce of fat was allowed on his body. Elizabeth continued smoking, and what he lost in weight, she gained. And, as before, she continued clubbing, when her job allowed. Chris simply couldn't understand how his partner's unfit body could bear a child without risk.

Meanwhile, Elizabeth seemed to be unable to even hear the word "gym" and would have much rather carried on as before. Back then they had spent time together, gone to parties, loved each other, seen movies, frittered away Sundays in bed, and smoked. She found it difficult that Chris had become a loner while she still enjoyed going out with people.

Now I wanted to know from Chris what he needed from the partnership that was missing.

His answer: "That she get off her butt and go swimming with me, or that we take a trip down the river or go to an exhibition." Hadn't both of them said something about love? There it was. "We wouldn't dream of splitting up. We love each other too much." I had the suspicion that their concept of love had a few fractures.

One month later Chris came to the office alone.

"It really upsets me how Elizabeth treats her body," he admitted again. "It turns me right off." He scoffed at her weakness in not being able to quit smoking or drinking. But Chris wasn't only worried about his and Elizabeth's health: he was on the verge of turning into a health fanatic. Other ways of life, different from his own, were unacceptable. There was no trace in him of understanding or a hint of lenience. The longer he argued his philosophy, the more annoyed he became at the thought that he and a woman like Elizabeth were together and planning on having kids.

I had already had in my practice a number of couples in which one partner suffered because the other smoked. Smoking is definitely a reason for breakups.

"And has smoking had an impact on sex?" I asked.

Chris nodded. "Everything about Elizabeth stinks of smoke—her hair, every single pore of her body."

Finally he got down to talking about his penis's erection problem, which Elizabeth had already addressed in the joint session.

"How do you masturbate?" I wanted to know. "How exactly do you arouse yourself?"

"I lie in bed when Elizabeth is on her night shift, or do it in the shower. It takes a minute or two."

Chris's masturbation involved a high level of tension, and he came quickly. Again, there was obviously more need than pleasure involved. I then asked him to describe his fantasies: whatever the imagination dreams up to turn someone on is usually a reflection of their own sexual system. In his little "head movies," Chris was surrounded by women. Sexual intercourse wasn't paramount, but when it did occur, it was, in his mind, always another man performing and not him. He enjoyed being touched by women he didn't have to look at and who also avoided looking him in the eye. He was only interested in looking at breasts and, as he put it, "pussies." He wanted to lick everything. What he wanted most of all was to be given fellatio by the women, but Elizabeth didn't like performing oral sex.

"I never think of Elizabeth when I do it myself," he concluded, "and that makes me sad."

At the end of the session I asked him how well or badly the relationship was going. "Five to twelve or five past twelve?"

"Eleven forty-five," answered Chris. Well, there was some hope, then.

That didn't sound so bad—better than I expected. He would be happy, he continued, if Elizabeth would begin by changing her mindset. For his plans in life, his desire to start a family, he needed someone who was pulling in the same direction—preferably Elizabeth, but a reformed Elizabeth. What kind of logic is that?

The two of them, I reflected, were at a stalemate and both unable to act. Every possible solution would seem equally good or equally bad and would only make the stalemate more resolute. For a while an artificial balance like that could be maintained, but in the long term it couldn't turn out well. Chris and Elizabeth would have to shift; pressure on them had to be increased. And they were going to have to acknowledge that their love, in this crippling situation, was to some extent deceit. I decided that it would be my task in the next session to break through these obstacles.

Two months passed before they both appeared again in my office. They explained that the situation had become more tense. Elizabeth was still smoking, and was still just as reluctant to take up some sport or other. And they hadn't had any sex, either. But at least she had stopped drinking, and she was working the day shift, so it wasn't as if she hadn't changed at all. But she wanted Chris to do more in the apartment, which he found difficult as there was very little time left after all his athletic activities.

Chris was still convinced that he wanted to stay with Elizabeth—she just had to comply with his wishes. It was damn tricky.

"Would separation be an option?" I asked directly.

Chris needed no time to reply: "Definitely not!"

"I still think Chris is great and sexy." Elizabeth's reply also wasn't particularly hesitant.

Despite all assurances and acknowledgments, both were unhappy, especially Elizabeth, who felt she was being constantly bombarded with criticisms old and new. When Chris was out of the apartment, she whispered to me once on departing, she would make a grab for her pack of cigarettes, but with every cigarette she smoked, she was plagued by guilt. It was an endless struggle fought deep inside her. Instead of sex, togetherness, and affection, they had to cope with arguments from their partner. There was nothing positive, nothing Chris wanted and could suitably formulate. I could recognize no concessions on his part. I seriously feared that their relationship was at an end. And it would not be long before they too realized it . . . or some pivotal change took place—but what?

"But we're still *so* in love." This statement sometimes seems to me to be a death knell.

Another two months and everything between them seemed to be remarkably good—but then again not. They spoke much more intimately, and through this I got to hear that they were having sex again, even twice a week. Chris's problem with his erection seemed to have been resolved. The smoking problem was still a stumbling block, as was, in Elizabeth's opinion, the amount of time Chris spent on physical activity.

Their expectations of each other were still wide apart. They were drifting apart not because of lack of love but rather because of contrasting lifestyles. Chris's eyes lit up when he talked about his fitness and Elizabeth's when she talked about going out with her friends—she had remained the night owl she had been when she fell in love with Chris. She said that darkness was her home, where she could express her character, where she was full of energy. It would go against her nature to adopt Chris's regimen. No surprise, then, that she felt out of place at his side. Yet they were, as ever, unwilling to go their separate ways.

Love and sex have the dynamics of an elastic band. Sometimes everything is fine and life is bubbly, but then it can become quiet and slack. Maybe it's because something at work takes precedence, or building a house, or sick parents, or one's own health. Love, in these instances, is not so lively and fulfilling; sex doesn't have the same importance as at other times. These dynamics are totally understandable, and as long as they don't trigger fear, and people don't suddenly think that they have the wrong partner or that there's something wrong with the relationship, then everything is okay. Such couples are, according to Schnarch, adequately differentiated. Beneath everything there's certainty and confidence that love is still there and will soon glow again.

Love first begins to manifest itself as love when problems arise that need to be treated in an open, tolerant way. A love that is lived is more than the yearning for love shown in romantic movies, which is why most of those movies end in a kiss and "lived" love isn't even shown. In romantic love, you don't want to know about difficulties. And it was a little like this with Chris and Elizabeth. They were so caught up with their idea of love that they weren't able to see their difficulties in day-to-day life.

It was supposed to be their last session, on a hot summer's day slowly turning into a balmy evening—not an everyday occurrence in Hamburg. Once again, they had noted a number of improvements. Chris was now helping with the household chores. They were spending a lot of time with each other and were about to go on vacation. I advised them to plan to spend their time during these weeks as they each wanted, without bending to the other's wishes. The thought behind this was to make it clear to them during that time how different their interests still were. Then maybe they could discover if splitting up would be the better option or if it made sense to maintain the relationship.

WHEN TO GO, WHEN TO STAY

Together we drew up a list of activities like "She goes out" and "He goes jogging"—each telling the other how many of these activities could be tolerated by the other in their daily life (also considering time on vacation together) and how much was necessary for their own well-being. Chris wrote, "Elizabeth going out—once or twice a month." On Elizabeth's note: "Chris jogging—once a week, sometimes twice." Once more they could see the distance between their expectations.

I tried to get to the point about the ramifications: "How about more or less stopping training, Chris?" And then to his partner: "Or completely giving up going out, Elizabeth?" And then, after a short dramatic pause, the third possibility: "Or splitting up?" Only then did they realize that there were no other options. They understood that they lived with an idea of their relationship that was far removed from reality, and they were shocked. Both remained silent.

To differentiate and mature can hurt, as it is difficult to let the other person be different but still be there. To break away from symbiosis or another form of security, to free yourself from mutual use or abuse, can initially rouse feelings of loneliness, of being wronged or abandoned. The later gains, however, are great—feelings of joy, freedom, new energy, connection, and life.

I then told them about my separation from Peter and how we decided to carry on loving each other . . . and had continued to do so. I floated that story to show that there were alternatives, to indicate that splitting up doesn't necessarily mean cutting all ties to each other. What I had gathered from recent sessions was that they were very fond of each other as people.

I said to Chris and Elizabeth on parting, "Maybe you'll make it. You now know more about each other and what your situation is."

Their next and last appointment was supposed to be four weeks from then, after they got back from their vacation. Then I received this email:

> *Dear Ms. Henning,*
> *We no longer can/have to/may/need to keep our appoint-*
> *ment with you tomorrow. In brief, we have decided to split*
> *up. We spent a lot of time thinking things over, and we*
> *now believe that by breaking up, we have a chance of being*
> *happy in the long term. Together, however, no chance. Of*
> *course, it's very sad and we have difficult times in front of us,*
> *but we'll survive. Many thanks to you, even though it didn't*
> *turn out the way we all certainly hoped for at the beginning,*
> *but still, we came to a decision.*

Sometimes it's good to do what has to be done. It's never too late to change your direction in life.

Meaningful Endurance

IN MUCH THE same way, it's sometimes worth it to hang on and work on the relationship by focusing on differentiation —providing both partners are prepared to do so. An example: Sometimes I get mad at my current partner. We quarrel and I get annoyed, and he just stays silent and doesn't adopt a clear stance. On noticing that I'm criticizing him and want to argue with him, he just clams up. In my eyes, that's a weakness, a lack of resistance I don't suffer from. He sees things from a different perspective, one he first experienced as a child, namely, that if he defends himself, it's highly likely that he'll be severely reprimanded. He comes from a different culture from me, from a Latin American country where, unlike where he and I live now, children generally obey parents without question. This explains why it makes no sense for him to disagree with me or defend himself.

That he now does so is a sign of major progress for both of us, but it was hard work. We both suffered—and laughed. It was and sometimes still is an enormous strain. It takes me a lot of effort to put up with his reserve, with his placid face. I'm missing an opponent (although someone who says nothing, in doing so, is also saying something!). Sure, I usually leave him in peace with his reticence, but sometimes I insist on his presence, and then he just has to bite the bullet. There was a seemingly endless flux for us between symbiosis and differentiation, and at times we were on the verge of splitting up. But when I feel that there's momentum in the relationship, that we're more gentle with each other's weaknesses and are still developing as a couple, I realize that my partner's silences don't irritate me as much as they used to. He, for his part, has learned that sometimes it's worth stating an opinion. So, it still makes sense to persevere, to wait and see. This means working on differentiation, and it must be done—only then will the relationship remain alive.

This also helps me in my practice. The better I know myself, understand my relationship, and communicate with my partner, the more effective I become as a therapist. For certain I'm not someone who avoids tension, and not someone who chooses peace at the expense of discovery— neither privately, nor in the practice of love!

Like a Five-Year-Old

THE REWARDS OF working on differentiation were also felt by Franz and Helen. Do you remember the senior physician who wanted to know what I hadn't understood about his email?

I requested an appointment with the two of them, although his plan had been to send only his wife. I countered with, "You think only your wife has a problem. We may find out today that that's true—but maybe you're wrong."

My retort showed him that I was willing to withstand unpleasant situations and still hold a mirror up to him. And it was just this that was crucial to the course of the therapy.

Franz and Helen had been married for three years and, as Helen explained during her initial, individual session, had been trying to have a child for the past two. And because ovulation had occurred the day before, she had also talked about sex, which was, as always at that time, obligatory. They cuddled and kissed for hours, and it had been good sex. A short flashback:

"Franz was inside me for a long time, even after he fell asleep." At that time in their daily routine they were very close—it was true love between them; they felt at ease. What an ideal picture Helen was painting!

"But I don't know if he thinks I'm really hot, just that he loves me," she said, and this sentence seemed to jog her memory, because in the minutes that followed she flew into a rage. All of a sudden the beautiful pretense was smashed. Franz often kowtowed to people and was insecure, especially in front of his parents, and that's not at all sexy. He needed plenty of support: everything had to be the best, the biggest, the most beautiful. "He has enough stress for three people!" And sex with him was generally also a problem. Because of *his* wanting children, *she* felt like a rabbit. For instance, the last time they had sex, she would have liked to have come, but he, as usual, hadn't even noticed. She hadn't had an orgasm for over a year. Sometimes he was just too rough; his penis was too large, and once she even had to vomit when performing oral sex.

When Franz came with her to the second session, somewhat unwillingly, he also talked about his unfulfilled desire to have children. His wife had, years earlier, been to the doctor and discovered that without medical assistance, she probably wouldn't become pregnant. As a result, they had visited a fertility center and had found a clinic they trusted. They had been trying now for two years, but Helen was still not pregnant and often cried. She was having trouble bearing it, and the hormones she was prescribed made her bloated and touchy; she generally didn't feel good taking them. Franz expected her to initiate copious sex with him without thinking about "making children," despite his desire for them. He wanted "three hours of petting," Helen was to return to these three hours again and again, often saying, "He can have the sex, but not the three hours."

So there were a number of problems between her and Franz. What was important here, however, was the latent anger and how they argued.

Many couples try to hide their negative feelings in my office. But sometimes their anger is so great that it can no longer be contained. I have seen women totally dismantle their partners in their very presence.

Back to Franz and Helen. He sat down first. She commented on his behavior: "So, you're already sitting. As always, the best seat." She was smiling, it's true, but the word "always" got right to me. I envisaged a voodoo doll with a red needle stuck in its head, forcing someone, somewhere, into submission. And Franz knew that the needling with the "best seat" was just the beginning.

Still they professed:

"I love him more than anything in the world!"

"I love her too!"

I tried to explain: "You don't love each other more than anything in the world—if that were the case, you would stop being stubborn, be brave, and really try to change things and behave differently."

Anyway, Helen and Franz quarreled so much and so loudly during their first couples session that toward the end I had to mention it. "For ninety minutes I've had to witness you verbally mistreat each other. As far as I'm concerned, you're free to do that at home, but not here. You certainly don't want to pay just so I can watch this drama, do you?" Both shook their heads and considered my intervention reasonable.

The crucial scene with Helen and Franz took place in the fourth session, as they both were hollering at the tops of their lungs (no, I couldn't stop them). After many mutual accusations—they seemed like squabbling siblings—I abruptly interrupted them, stared directly at Franz, and said, "I have a very serious question for you." Out of the corner of my eye I saw Helen grin. She seemed to think it was good that her husband was about to get a serious dressing down. Without looking at her, I continued: "And I am well aware that Helen is sitting there finding all this very amusing, although it's not at all funny for either of you." Helen immediately felt exposed and her expression changed. I continued: "How old, normally, is someone who behaves like you've been behaving for the last half hour? What do you think?" I kept my eyes firmly on him. He was attentive.

Franz's answer was plain: "Five."

I nodded. What followed can be explained quickly. Franz was now perfectly calm. My remarks about his behavior had turned his image of himself upside down. Eventually, he said he didn't want to be a childish man. He accepted my criticism without further ado, and lo and behold, Helen immediately felt a change in his conduct. At the end of the meeting, when her husband made a short visit to the men's room, Helen looked at me with surprise in her eyes: "Well, well, well. I've never seen him like that before! Somehow I think that's really hot . . ." No doubt about it, Franz proved he had some style and standing!

8

The Lanzarote Effect:

THE CHILD IN ADULT RELATIONSHIPS

U P TO THIS point I have described the standard concepts of love rather than put those concepts on a pedestal. But I hope that I've made it clear how deeply I believe in love and how indispensable it is to life. Love can heal; it allows us to grow, and sometimes it just feels wonderful. Why then are there so many problems with it? Because love means bonding, and bonding, in turn, doesn't always trigger positive feelings. "People are creatures of relationship who are programmed to bond and whose chances of survival depend on fulfilling their existential basic needs for acceptance and belonging," wrote the renowned German sexologists Kurt Loewit and Klaus M. Beier. Creatures of relationship! A super phrase that actually says everything. People are creatures who need and want relationships. That yearning is firmly fixed in our brains, so firmly that when our relationships start to wobble, we are frightened or hurt. Loewit and Beier continue: "We're talking about basic needs that become particularly marked in the physical closeness of (intimate) relationships—with the resulting feelings of comfort and security." If we experience these feelings, relationships are positive and invigorating. But cruelty, disgust (see the story of Shayne and his mother), or the fear of losing someone can cause strong negative relationships and activate symbiotic processes.

In the worst cases, we are no longer able to free ourselves from these negative bonds—our emotional dependence is too powerful. There is, at the beginning of every human life, perfect symbiosis; that is to say, when we are in our mother's womb, we have an all-encompassing feeling of security. In the first years of infancy, the symbiotic relationships with parents and other family members are of enormous, even existential, importance; without them we simply couldn't survive. The child is dependent on these people's unconditional love, and clings to them, in a positive way. After some time, however, a child wants to escape all that and, full of expectation, to discover the world, get to know their own abilities, and explore the possibilities of independence. Of course they always return to their loved ones—for reassurance, comfort, and security—and in doing so, they reaffirm some kind of basic trust. At some point, however, every child *doesn't* get what he or she wants. The parents refuse something or other, set limits. Or the parents, for whatever reason, are not there to hug or cosset the child at a crucial moment. At first this experience is traumatic for a child. Children then feel frightened and angry. Up until then, everything has been based on *them,* and now, all of a sudden, they are no longer the center of attention. But one single moment of uncertainty doesn't have to become a full drama; such moments are part of the normal development process. They become a problem only if the stress becomes permanent and if needs are constantly ignored. This provokes anger, which in turn causes feelings of guilt and of anxiety that something similar could happen again. Then, often, suppression kicks in and prevents the development of the basic social and cognitive capabilities that everyone ultimately needs for a satisfying life.

Everyone knows the kids at the supermarket checkout who don't get candy they really want. They throw themselves to the ground, thrashing around and screaming their heads off. They're angry, and at that moment they hate their mothers. Let's call it "murderous rage." Do you recognize the scene? Then let's venture a little mind game: Imagine that kid now as a twenty-one-year-old with a knife in his hand. Can you feel the hate? The stubborn kid at the checkout was, fortunately, just a few feet tall, and his anger at his mother scared him, as he knew (subconsciously) that he was dependent on her. His mother's reaction to his behavior at this difficult moment was of immense importance. Does she lovingly guide the child through the experience (even when he didn't get the candy), does she punish him by ignoring the situation for either a brief or longer period, or does she start shouting at him? Over time children's black-and-white world turns gray. The child discovers that conflicts with their nearest and dearest don't mean separation or the withdrawal of love. At some point they come to understand that love tolerates, that two people can have their own opinions. Little by little, they then learn to let go of the comfort and security of a symbiotic relationship and to take care of themselves. At the latest, when a person has grown up, symbiosis—the very close bonding in which someone is too dependent on someone else—should be over.

But, you might think, it was so great at that time, when someone else was devotedly and lovingly taking care of you —it was so warm and cozy, so carefree! And you'd be right.

Precisely for this reason we continue to look back—and to fall in love. Being in love is symbiotic superglue! There they are again, comforting feelings of times gone by. Someone else wants only *me!* I glow and blossom: he's doing everything in his power just to see me; he acknowledges me all the time, and vice versa. We marvel at each other. If doubts begin to emerge, they are shunted to the side. We feel adopted and adapted to by our lover. The world around us can cause us no harm.

So what's the problem? There isn't one, at least not as long as we're in love. Love becomes a "danger" only when we take off our rose-colored glasses, when we are challenged, when we are denied something, and when new limits are set—exactly as it was for us with our parents.

Love reminds us of what was once good but also of fears of being rejected or abandoned. The first shock was written all over our faces long ago when we crawled up to Mom only to realize she had no time for us, and that feeling still sits deep in us. This is also why many adults don't manage to become independent beings, why they are highly emotional and symbiotic in relationships, are dependent on their partners and have difficulty being themselves. They are missing the positive aspects of distance and its place in their lives.

In our close relationships, when we are in love, our childhood is switched on. And a lot of people had childhoods that you wouldn't describe as happy. The conditions for developing into a self-confident person who is responsible for their own actions do not always occur early on. Early troubles—especially in relationships with the people in our inner circle—leave deep marks on us, and to a certain extent determine our love lives later. Parents don't want to let go, and we don't want to go.

In practical therapy, we're often dealing with abandoning these strong ties—ties to a partner and very often also to parents. Clients are sometimes amazed: "Why on earth should I distance myself from my parents? I never ask them for advice. I live my own life." On looking closer, however, it's not always necessary to ask parents for advice; even without contact, they're making decisions for you. The client knows, consciously or subconsciously, what their parents are like, how they support or deny them, and often act accordingly . . . even as adults. Particularly when dealing with sexual issues, this is often of huge significance.

Shame, moral or emotional constraints . . . It cannot be stressed too strongly how much we are influenced by our parents' ideas and values—and by their fears.

All this is normal, but as long as we nurture strong symbiotic feelings toward our parents, it will be difficult to develop our own concepts of life and love. Some clients, like sleepwalkers or people under hypnosis, don't realize how blindly their patterns follow their childhood. This becomes more obvious when clients have long felt that they have very different opinions from their parents but they still can't manage to assert themselves or change their own lives. Time and again they don't stand up for themselves. And the more symbiotic our links, the harder they are to loosen.

Hence, in the practice of love, the task is often to try to shake off the constraints we were given as kids that do not allow us to govern our lives. We adults need to find a healthy balance between autonomy and symbiosis, both in relation to our parents and in relation to our partners.

Lucky Swine

HERE AND THERE in my office are a couple of cute eye-catchers, such as my little copper pig sleeping soundly on a cushion. There was quite a domestic tussle when I saw it in the store window and wanted to buy it. Although I had my own income, my husband was against buying it—far too expensive, you can't possibly pay *that* much for a copper pig (and yes, it was pricey). At that time, I thought I had to get my own way by quarreling. I was making my husband's problem *my* problem: very symbiotic. Today I don't ask anyone if I want to buy or do something. I just do it, without any ado. The little copper pig has now become a symbol of my development—a differentiation pig! As if my clients can smell it, almost all of them comment on it—how peacefully it's sleeping. Yup! Differentiation makes you happy.

Love in the Brain

A FAMOUS NEUROLOGIST and psychologist wrote to Albert Einstein at the beginning of the twentieth century, "We must recollect that all our provisional ideas in psychology will presumably some-day be based on an organic substructure. This makes it probable that it is special substances and chemical processes which perform the operations of sexuality and provide for the extension of individual life into that of the species."

It was Sigmund Freud.

Almost a century later the British DNA researcher and Nobel Prize winner Francis Crick said much the same at a conference: "You, your joys, and your sorrows, your memories and ambitions, your sense of personal identity and freewill, are in fact no more than the behavior of a vast assembly of nerve cells and their associated molecules."

And at this point once again my pragmatism pipes up. For me as a sexologist, that pragmatism means I am convinced that we can and must talk about sex and love in scientific terms. This doesn't fit many people's romantic concepts, but sex and love are also biochemical processes. They make us blind and in love for six days or six weeks—and then the next twenty-five years begin.

Our feelings are biochemical processes that react to what's happening around us. If we are sad, that could mean that splitting up is imminent. If we are angry, the message could be "Let's get the hell out of here!" or "Attack!" These sentiments are triggered by neurotransmitters, dopamine or adrenaline, which are responsible for transmission of signals from one nerve cell to the other.

While studying neuropsychology, I began to understand how flexible and obstinate the brain is. About 5 percent of its decisions are deliberately controlled by us—we're talking conscious processes here. The vast majority of processes in the brain, however, happen subconsciously, without our knowledge. Consciousness versus subconsciousness: how do they interact? Could the subconscious be our most important sensory organ? Freud, the man who popularized the subconscious (which he often interchangeably referred to as the "unconscious"), was of the opinion that it was, rather, the enemy. Today many people disagree with this point of view and see the subconscious more as a friend without which we would be unable to cope with day-to-day life.

Many scientists research consciousness, including the American cell and developmental biologist Bruce Lipton. Lipton has described how the conscious mind functions deliberately, sets objectives, and is constantly making judgments while also always trying out something new. It is creative but can perform no more than three activities at any given moment and uses only short-term memory for storage. It deals with some two thousand pieces of information per second, one after the other—the past, present, and future all exist in our conscious minds. Our consciousness is aware of what has just happened and what will happen next.

The subconscious mind, on the other hand, has no such sense of time; it really couldn't care less whether something has just taken place or is about to—for the subconscious, everything is happening right now. Luckily, this part of our brains has further processing capabilities: thousands of activities (breathing, heartbeat, blood pressure, temperature perception, digestion, and so on) can be simultaneously executed and analyzed—on average four billion pieces of information per second. So while the 5 percent of our mind that is conscious is constantly (slowly) thinking, the 95 percent that is subconscious is running the show. The bottom line is this: the subconscious mind governs our behavior.

The power of the subconscious, the forces that it releases in the depths of our egos, left a lasting impression on me, the consequences of which crop up daily in my practice. Oh yes, and I almost forgot: the subconscious doesn't like anything new. In no way is it curious. Everything should remain as it was—no changes, please. And this: it remembers everything...especially things that hurt. It has to.

Nothing Is Forgotten

IN THE HUMAN brain is a warning system whose only job is to keep us alive. It is one of the oldest parts of our brains: it developed around 500 million years ago. This warning mechanism is part of our limbic system, the hub of all our emotions, deep within our brains. Phylogenetically, it is thought to have evolved during the transition from reptilian brain to early mammalian brain. Our warning systems react instantly, quasi-automatically; they are independent of conscious thought and are always in the "now" mode; they are always wide awake. This is our fight-or-flight response mechanism, and it takes command in situations of stress or anxiety, telling us that we are dealing not with a harmless deer but with a ravenous wolf. Although (or because) the system is ancient, it is still extremely powerful.

The limbic system's components include the amygdala (from the Latin word for "almond"), one in each temporal lobe, and the hippocampus (named after its resemblance to a seahorse), of which there are also two. Both components —the amygdala, responsible for warnings, and the hippocampus, responsible for memory—are involved in the beginnings of fear in the context of situations and, linked to this, in recognizing these situations and their possible dangers. Interestingly, the amygdala also seems to be involved in sensing all forms of arousal, including sexual.

This too is important: Our warning system learns from experience, starting at birth. Whether we find something pleasant or unpleasant, harmful or harmless depends on what we link it to—perceptions are reconstructions. Every adventure, every experience we have, is compared to everything we have ever experienced and stored. Only then can we decide: harmful or harmless? Pleasant or unpleasant? This is why our memory, our past, is so important to us.

There is another important team player in the system: the insular cortex. This is located deep inside the hemispheres of the cerebral cortex, is closely linked to the amygdala and hippocampus, acts as the command center for all forms of arousal, and regulates all basic emotions. It also plays a huge role in homeostasis—the body's equilibrium, such as telling us when our bladder is full, how to assess pain, and to get ready for an orgasm. The insular cortex is particularly active when situations exceed the norm or cross boundaries, and is linked to mind mapping—so here begins disgust. All in all, the little watchdogs in our brains have quite a lot to do with sexuality.

However, after traumatic experiences, there can be enormous strain on the psyche, and memory can fail. For example, people who have been sexually assaulted sometimes can't consciously remember what has happened to them. The ordeal stored in the subconscious is not accessible, which provides protection against feelings like shame, disgust, shock, or even guilt. Shayne couldn't perceive the abuse by his mother as a part of his own personality, as part of his own past. The truth, how cruelly he had been treated by his own mother, would have been too much of a burden for him. His brain's trick was to declare the experience nonexistent, a no-go area.

"I've Always Done It That Way"

SOMETIMES MAKING A decisive step toward splitting up just feels impossible. Even finally telling your partner precisely what you think can feel that way, or changing something about a relationship and heading for terra incognita. Neurologically, this is down to the fact that the subconscious does *not* like anything it doesn't already know. Things unfamiliar are rigorously quashed; the subconscious would rather stick to recognized patterns, however bad those might be.

This is why habits are pretty much like natural laws. With the help of habits, we can cope with a lot of things, maybe even almost everything. Habits are the path of least resistance, and it takes a long time for new courses of actions to break old routines. Habits develop because they work, and are retained because they will continue to function in the future. And you already aren't telling your partner what you think about bad sex and what you would *really* like to try instead. Rather, it's business as usual: persisting with old models induces less anxiety and saves time and energy. Therapy means breaking these patterns, and breaking them is going to feel like hard work.

Lanzarote

TO ILLUSTRATE TO my clients the two main features of our subconscious ("I remember everything" and "I don't like anything new"), I sometimes tell them about an experience I once had on Lanzarote in the Canary Islands. I was vacationing with my husband and our son on the volcanic island. In our hotel we found a brochure about Lanzarote's many underground lava caves and lakes, which were formed between 3,000 and 4,500 years ago. We booked a tour after reading that the inhabitants apparently hid there from pirates, which we thought would interest our son.

After passing through a narrow passage in the cliff face to enter the cave system, the first thing I noticed was a lake behind a red-and-white-striped tape that spanned the cave. The cave was illuminated by a number of small lamps that hinted at the lake's great depth. The water was so clear that my son and I could look deep into the crater. The lake walls were rough, and the deeper they went, the darker they became. My husband remained near the rear wall of the cave, as far away from the lake as possible—he was frightened of heights and depths. I could understand him: the place felt oppressive.

When all the visitors had gathered and were whispering behind the tape, the guide stressed how deep the ancient lake was—as if that was necessary. Then he calmly took a small pebble out of his pocket and tossed it into the lake. *Ha!* I thought. *He sure knows how to frighten naive tourists.* And also how to trick them. The pebble didn't sink into the endless depths of a bottomless lake but bounced with a sharp crack on the floor of a two-inch puddle. And then I got it—the impression of depth came solely from the reflection of the cave roof on the surface of the water. As a grand finale, the guide, with a flourish of his hand and a smile, ripped away the tape and said, "Five dollars to anyone who jumps in!"

I then knew that in front of me there wasn't a deep lake, not even a pond, but a ridiculous puddle. However, after the ripples from the pebble had slowly disappeared, the reflection once again gave the impression of incredible depth. So clear was the reflection that you didn't notice the water, only the crater. The guide said to me, "Go on, jump!"

My consciousness tried: *Go on, the water's not deep. It's a trick!* I knelt down and, heart pounding, bent forward to touch the bottom with my hand. I found that the bottom really was just a hand's width down. I stood up and, with a great effort, dipped the tip of my toe into the water. (I was wearing flip-flops.) The same result: I could touch the bottom. The guide, who still had his eyes on me, said, "Go for it! Just jump!"

I tried, but I couldn't! I was doubly sure that it was shallow, but still the subconscious said *No!* Maybe it would have been possible to go in step by step, although I'm still not sure I could have done it. But the command was: "Jump!"

The end of the story: the guide kept his five dollars. He had successfully managed to play with our primal fears and our subconscious.

This story illustrates to my clients why it is so difficult to change patterns when fears are involved. They feel confirmation that the change about to happen in their lives is not going to be easy, no piece of cake. In fact, it will be more like learning to play the violin. You practice a lot, and you simply have to start somewhere. If a client who knows the cave story comes to me a bit down and complains about how long it takes to make progress (and sometimes my clients are very hard on themselves), I just say, "Lanzarote."

9

Shutdown:

WHEN LEGS
ARE CROSSED

HOW SEXUALITY DEVELOPS and how relationship patterns take shape have, as I have pointed out, a lot to do with our experiences as children. Children, when playing with others, practice showing feelings, communicating, experiencing happiness and pleasure. Parents take care of us physically—they hold us and stroke us—but in the end we all get to know our bodies ourselves. Childishly, playfully, and with plenty of curiosity, we enjoy the rewards of these amazing and exciting experiences. For instance, boys quickly discover that something is dangling down there, and generally there's nothing to stop them from doing a bit of leisurely research. For girls things are slightly different, as it's considerably more difficult to build up a positive relationship with what's "down there," but doing so is particularly important for a girl's positive relationship with her own sexuality, for her as a sexual being.

Female clients in particular often describe experiences from their childhood and adolescence that had a negative influence on their development into sexually confident women—maybe struggles with fathers, brothers, uncles, or grandfathers who crossed boundaries. Often, prudish or even anti-sex mothers or grandmothers punished their daughter or granddaughter for her early spirit of discovery. This makes it difficult for these women to have the love life they would like to as adults. What follows is about these women.

Naked Dancing

JENNIFER—LARGE, MID-THIRTIES, married—came to the practice with a problem in which her childhood had an important role: she suffered from vaginismus. This condition is the result of an involuntary vaginal muscle spasm and some of the surrounding pelvic floor muscles making the vagina too narrow or even completely closing it.

The client told me about an experience she had had as a seven-year-old. Happy as a clam, she was in the tub playing with her rubber duck. Afterward she danced around the bathroom singing happily, looking at her own naked movements in the mirror. Then her mother passed by: the door was open, and she saw her daughter naked and chirpy. She rushed in immediately, grabbing Jennifer so hard by the arm that she left bruises. Half an hour later they were sitting at the big kitchen table. There was death silence. The family said nothing. Jennifer's two elder sisters, her brother, her mother, of course, and her father—all of them seemed to already know what had happened. Jennifer could read it in their stony faces. The punishment took place over several days and included rejection and neglect. No beating, no words of outrage—in fact, just the opposite. The little girl just had to *look* at her mother to feel guilty. This is how negative associations come into being. A child wishes to please their mother but receives no acknowledgment, no recognition, so they try even harder and become even more emotionally dependent on her than they already were.

Jennifer's experience in front of the mirror was not the only one of its kind. Her parents' inability to countenance any forms of pleasure also affected her siblings. During love scenes in movies, the mother would literally throw herself in front of her children to protect them from "filth," or would suddenly turn the TV off if she thought that a kiss was about to happen. The result was that the dancing girl, Jennifer, became anorexic in puberty and developed a general aversion to sex.

During her first session Jennifer told me that although she had sexual desires for her husband, she somehow couldn't quite hide her feeling that she was being raped. "Someone is trying to get inside me—I don't like it!" She would, however, dearly love to be a mother. She had a desperate yearning for motherhood, almost as if her life depended on it. She thought that with a child, everything would be better.

When it comes to traumatic childhood experiences, it's very important during therapy to help the client pragmatically recognize what their parents were really like and not merely defend the parents' actions. Clients tread carefully, symbiotically protecting their parents, and then have trouble getting on in life; this cannot be my approach as a therapist. Instead, I try to get as accurate a picture of the situation at that time as possible, as if I had a camera and could zoom in on certain aspects. There are close-ups of all the faces, and I listen solemnly to the movie director giving instructions, to the client telling me who felt what toward whom. The director, of course, is always the client—in this case, Jennifer, who had to describe the feelings of all those sitting at the kitchen table as if it were a scene from a movie. In this way, I could get not only information about all those present and who said what, but also a sense or inkling of what it must have felt like to be at that table in that moment.

In Jennifer's case, the crushing silence at the evening meal was a key piece of information. Had I seen this scene merely as a silent punishment, I might have come to the conclusion that while it was certainly an unpleasant situation, the damage was within acceptable limits. But going into detail with the client and learning what each member of that family felt about imagining a naked Jennifer—and all this in a family where nakedness was forbidden and considered a crime—the client could feel how great the impact was at that time and how great the shame (and so could I): great enough for Jennifer to begin to reject a body capable of enjoying such "filthy" feelings as the freedom of nudity. On further questioning from me about other situations, there would probably be even more to fill out the picture—maybe her sisters' and brother's schadenfreude, their satisfaction that someone else was worse off than them. Jennifer's experience had taken place thirty years earlier, yet her memories were crystal clear. Just think about it! What had the little girl done wrong? Absolutely nothing!

By looking back, clients can gain a realistic understanding of their situation and can finally see their parents' cruelty, maybe indifference, or even sexual motivation. It's a crazy world in which the brutal or cruel get a small dose of dopamine—our brain's reward system is stimulated by such acts. Generally, dopamine is present at the beginning of all desires; it motivates us, arouses us, including sexually (the insular cortex!). But in the realm of negative sexuality, I find the links between dopamine and the resulting behavior hardest to bear.

Even as an adult, Jennifer refused to accept her female body. She couldn't become pregnant, although she really wanted to, but not because her vaginismus left her unable to have sexual intercourse: even treatment in a fertility clinic had failed to have the desired effect. As she began to understand how her mother had mistreated her and her sisters, and as this blind spot gradually began to heal, other painful memories began to emerge.

Jennifer cried a lot and always tried to defend her mother until it was no longer possible or necessary. Finally, she could see the woman for what she was: evil and indifferent to the feelings of her children. And she understood that the situation never seemed important enough to her father for him to intervene and stop his wife. And yes, the fact that her mother grew up at a different time did mean that shame and guilt belonged for her among the basic tenets of parenting, especially for girls. Above all: "No sex (or sexual feelings) before marriage." Jennifer's mother had thoughtlessly passed down this moral straitjacket.

I managed to convince Jennifer to have a session with her parents in the sheltered confines of my office. Sometimes clients don't manage to hold such necessary clarifying talks with their parents by themselves. The aim, in the best-case scenario, is to try to loosen or break the symbiotic relationship with the parents. At family gatherings Jennifer had until then been quiet about the whole thing, and had avoided conflicts instead of confronting her parents with a few hard truths.

Her aggressive mother and apathetic father agreed to participate. In the discussion, Jennifer made clear that she had seen through the family's unhealthy dynamics, and the parents realized that now there were new boundaries. The discussion influenced the dynamics within the whole family. None of the family members had the hold over Jennifer that they'd previously had.

Clients bravely confront their parents only when they feel secure enough and can live with the consequences of this meeting no matter what those consequences are. They have confidence in themselves—a wonderful feeling!

It could have been sheer coincidence, but once Jennifer had freed herself from her strong, negative symbiotic ties to her mother, she became pregnant. She and her husband have now become parents and have decided within the small circle of their family to often dance naked in front of the mirror.

As I have already said, childhood is always present in relationships.

"You Will Be Drilled!"

"SOMEHOW I JUST never got around to it," Ricarda, a charming forty-one-year-old from Italy, tells me. She is evidently amazed herself, as her eyebrows arch, her shoulders hunch, and she gently shakes her head. She is talking about sexual intercourse. An aunt in Milan had once warned her, with an ominous expression, "Watch out! You will be drilled!" The advice came just after church, as Ricarda was about to be met outside for the first time by a boy from her school who was interested in her.

Another remark Ricarda remembered from her very religious upbringing was "Men are only interested in one thing. Save yourself for your husband." Later she was very nearly raped in a train. Her attacker held her arms above her head, pressing her against the wall of the carriage, talked about her "pussy," and kissed her roughly. As they were alone in the compartment, it was a dangerous situation. But Ricarda managed to defend herself and her attacker released her. That was when Ricarda decided that she didn't like men.

Eventually, however, she did get to know a man and they married. But they never had sexual intercourse and, like Jennifer, she had developed vaginismus. When I got to know her, she had already been divorced for ten years. She still was waiting for her penetrative sexual debut. She was becoming increasingly sad about this and had more than once considered suicide, but at the same time she was filled with an inner rage.

When after a number of therapy sessions Ricarda was showing signs of improvement, she found a new friend. She told me, full of optimism, that soon she would have her first experience of sexual intercourse—she was sure of it. Her inner readiness arose from her new partner not having insisted on intercourse: on the contrary, he had been lovingly restrained, and the "rest of sex" had been perfectly okay. Ricarda was feeling real desire. Both of them enjoyed heavy petting, but there had been no penetration.

You remember the gas pedal metaphor? Ricarda had a steady gas pedal. She didn't limit her desires even though she hadn't yet agreed to penetrative sex (being "drilled"!).

Transgressions or abuse, including sexual abuse, are not always physical. Clear dubious intentions and threatening, derogatory, or moralistic remarks from a close family member can cause serious damage. Ricarda had mapped the shamefaced, religious, anti-sex women in her family well: sex was dangerous!

Before coming to me with her vaginismus, Ricarda had had many appointments with her gynecologist. During these visits, she was terrified of lying on the examination table with her legs spread and of the pain from having the speculum and fingers inserted inside her. Every time she was there, she managed to terminate the check-up just in time—from her point of view.

As Ricarda didn't have the strength to try again, I called to get her an appointment with a different, well-known female gynecologist. When I phoned the office during our session and asked the receptionist whether it was possible to have an examination without the speculum, she answered firmly: "No. Why on earth should we? We always use that instrument." When I explained that my client suffered from vaginismus, she claimed never to have heard of it.

I thanked her and hung up.

Afterward I arranged an appointment for Ricarda with my own gynecologist. The examination took place without a speculum: it can be done just by external touch and ultrasound. The gynecologist had an understanding and knowledge of how patients with vaginismus feel.

Many women with vaginismus have experiences like Ricarda did with dismissive gynecologists. It's not uncommon for me to get emails from sufferers like Lisa:

> I (24 years old) suffered from vaginismus. Maybe not quite as dramatically as some other women—tampons were no problem (usually, anyway)—but sex was almost unthinkable, especially as after a couple of tries I always suffered from bladder infections. [Author's note: With a certain

amount of tension, it's not surprising that the urethra is affected.] As a result, I don't feel like sex in the first place. Two gynecologists just said, "You're slim-built. You just have to live with it." After the first session with a sex thera-pist, the vaginismus wasn't such a worry, as I knew that it's possible to cure it. So many women have to put up with this problem for years and don't find a solution, because many gynecologists have no idea that vaginismus exists. [Author's note: They also have no idea how to treat it, and it takes time that they do not have.] I didn't want to just accept that, so I approached my homeopath. She hadn't heard of vaginismus, but we put our heads together and researched what we could do about it. Among other things, the subject of my tense jaw cropped up. I began delving into progressive muscle relaxation. That was six months ago. Four weeks ago there was a breakthrough. I had sex with my partner—who, by the way, was very patient—and there was no pain.

Women like Lisa have vaginismus that still allows them to go to their gynecologist like normal and to use tampons without difficulties. (For this very reason, they are laughed at when they talk about their issues.) Their problems with sexual intercourse, however, remain.

Women Who Don't Want to Grow Up

"I SUFFER FROM vaginismus!" Katrina's ponytail swung back and forth as she sat down in the armchair. The twenty-nine-year-old sat there with her pelvis jutting forward and her legs slightly apart, and had she not been wearing jeans, I would have had a direct view of her crotch. Already after a few minutes I had the impression that Katrina behaved like a little girl who didn't have the slightest idea that there are intimate areas not meant to be held up for general viewing.

"So you say you have vaginismus. How do you know?" I asked.

"It's what my doctor told me." She looked at me expectantly.

"Could you describe how this vaginismus feels?"

"It's like a burning pain—everything cramps up. It happens as soon as my husband attempts penetration. As if he's breaking my hymen every time."

The feeling that the entrance to the vagina is blocked is fairly common for women with vaginismus. As we've seen, there are many causes for this. Usually the head of the penis (if not, even earlier, the thought of penetration) triggers the blockade, which is often linked to elements of fear or anxiety—for instance: *I had pain down there and sex sometimes hurt.* But also: *I'm frightened of becoming pregnant.* Because of these fears, "it" clamps up. The pelvic floor muscles tighten, rather like the feeling you get with cramps, or they remain tense. And already the next attempt at sexual intercourse is doomed from the outset to failure. The door inside is slammed shut.

Katrina had known her husband for fourteen years—it was a childhood love—and they had two children, aged one and three. A striking feature in her case was that not only did she experience pain during sexual intercourse, but her husband's penis, she later said, was very big, and he was clumsy and not particularly sensitive. Again and again an insecure, almost naive, concept about what it can mean to be female was noticeable in Katrina. These first impressions were boosted over the course of therapy, and the feeling of insecurity particularly applied to Katrina's identity as a mother.

Conventional medicine differentiates between primary and secondary vaginismus. With primary vaginismus, penetration is impossible from the start, as for Ricarda, who was frightened of being "drilled." With secondary vaginismus, penetration is no longer successful after a phase when it *had* been possible, as for Katrina, who had become pregnant the natural way.

Katrina, however, couldn't feel or see herself as a mother. She wanted to continue being a teenager, going clubbing, flirting, smooching, having fun—sometimes just for approval. But she never took things too far: she was much too scared of becoming pregnant again. Calmly and objectively but sometimes faltering, she explained: "Just before I was eighteen I moved into an apartment with my husband. I didn't have to work and could live one day at a time until our first daughter was born. At the beginning I thought it was exciting to have a child, but the reality was different. Instead of partying, I had to look after the little one. Then Emma, our second child, arrived. I hadn't used contraceptives, even though I'd already had enough of children after the first one. I became depressed, and was feeling so bad that I left my husband."

Since then, Katrina's husband had rejoined the family, and she was feeling better, though she was far from feeling full of life. Defensively, she continued: "I don't like my life as a mother. The girls are stealing everything from me. Without them life would be fun. Without them I wouldn't have responsibilities."

I wanted to know how long she had had vaginal tension.

"Roughly since the children were born."

"Do you still have sex with your husband?"

"When he rubs me, I get moist and aroused. Then we have sex without penetration. I refuse to take the pill, so it's better that way."

First of all, I recommended condoms. At roughly the same time as Katrina's problem was developing, however, her husband was diagnosed with phimosis, a condition in which the foreskin can't be pulled back over the glans. This made slipping on a condom almost impossible without pain. The phimosis was later operated on successfully, but at the time another solution had to be found. Waiving sex was one possibility; a closed vagina, the other.

A Narrow Tunnel, an Open Cave

THE SEX ORGAN as a source of femaleness or maleness seems archaic. But many women don't really believe how important for good sex it is to know and like your genitals, and instead perceive their femininity via their breasts or long hair. Yes, those are also important, but they aren't everything. If I compare women to men, the penny usually drops. "Have you ever had sex with a man who didn't really know or like his penis?" Should this not be enough, I follow up with "Have you ever had sex with a man who thought his penis was disgusting?" At this point at the latest, women agree to pay more attention to their own genitalia.

Genitals—and physicality in general—are particularly important for women with vaginismus. They often have false impressions of scale: in their mind, every penis is massive, every vagina small and narrow. It is hardly surprising that the idea of penetration is linked to worry and fear; this is actually quite normal and healthy.

Treating vaginismus is concerned, among other things, with adjusting to anatomic realities. This includes making the client aware of how flexible the vagina is—even a baby manages to pass through. I get women to draw the vulva, the external female sex organ, and talk about it before we, mentally, work our way inside.

"What does your vagina look like? What do you think of it?" I ask, and not only to Katrina.

"It's like a narrow tunnel!"

A typical answer for someone with vaginismus.

Many other women see their vaginas as caves, wide and open. With these clients I hold my finger in the air and say, "Do you feel anything in the cave?" I want them to realize how much pleasurable sensation is possible when the surroundings are empty space, not tissues. Usually there's no reply, so I continue: "Is it an airy feeling? Or more like a void?"

Sexologists, in this case, speak of an "uninhabited" vagina. Clients' perceptions gradually change once they know a little more. Visually, a vagina is like a flat glove: the entrance is softly sealed by tissue meeting tissue. It consists of a cylinder of surrounding tissue through which a finger or penis can easily penetrate. A penis, on sliding in, can normally open the vagina without any trouble.

While working with Katrina, I noticed her bodily reactions and saw how tension increased when certain subjects were discussed. "Have a feel. Did you notice how you just tensed your shoulders?"

Katrina had a feel. "Oh, yes! This is all so new for me ..."

She gulped, noticeably, a couple of times in a row, so I asked her to move parts of her upper body. There appeared to be some sort of emotional tension there. And I gave her a number of instructions: "Move your jaw," "Swivel your pelvis in small circles, as if you wanted to get a small bowl of marbles moving." Katrina seemed to be enjoying this. Her movements were calm and fluid even when she was sitting. "Take a deep breath—right down to your pelvis—and try to trace how you feel."

She did so. Her breath massaged all her organs. And with the movement, tension diminished. Katrina became more relaxed and even sensual.

Fleshlight

MANY WOMEN SUFFERING from vaginismus have an unusually limp handshake. It feels as if the hand, and with it the whole person, cannot be grasped, as if these clients, even when being greeted, are protecting themselves from some kind of energy penetration by retreating inside themselves. During a session we may practice firm handshaking, and I often discover how difficult this is for some clients.

I discovered another tool that I use in therapy—working with a fleshlight—by chance. A fleshlight is a kind of artificial silicon vagina embedded in a harder plastic shell. It looks like an oversized flashlight, hence the name. It's open at one end, and there's a screw cap at the other. It was originally intended for the penis. Men can masturbate with it with a certain sensation of reality, and I recommend it for thrusting exercises.

With the aid of a fleshlight, I wanted to simulate vaginismus for Katrina and to demonstrate, mainly for her own understanding, how she could try penetrating a fleshlight with a dildo. During therapy we tried it with gel, without gel, with a cap, and without one. In the course of this exercise, she was able to feel the difference in penetration, whether it was easy or difficult. When I unscrewed the cap, the air displaced by the dildo could escape; there was a feeling of expanse. When I screwed the cap on, the displaced air couldn't go anywhere, so things got tight in the artificial vagina, in much the same way as in a woman contracting her pelvic muscles around a penis.

We got down to work at once. I gathered a variety of dildos and some gel from my stocks. I really would have loved to have tried out the massive flesh-colored penis from the sex store—with bulging veins and other consistent anatomical details—but I wasn't sure whether it was too big for the rather narrow fleshlight. After Katrina and I managed to playfully introduce the smaller dildos with ease, we decided to try the big one. We smeared plenty of gel onto both it and the fleshlight to try to facilitate the seemingly impossible penetration. We even left the cap on to simulate a firm pelvic floor. And then? The monstrous penis slid in easily! I'm not sure who was more astonished. Eventually Katrina even felt comfortable enough to slide the penis in and out of the fleshlight herself, which in itself was a huge step for someone with vaginismus. Afterward Katrina said that she wanted to try doing it later on at home with her finger. Katrina's latest findings: "The vagina is really incredibly flexible!"

It was never necessary with Katrina to recommend conventional dilators—dildos with different size settings, from a pinky finger's width up to that of a normal penis. Dilators can be useful for treating women suffering from vaginismus. The sufferer can insert the dilator, starting with the smallest size and changing to the next size up once they've slowly become accustomed to the first. I don't particularly like this method; it's not organic enough for me. Dilators are like rods: smooth, cold, and unerotic, and they hardly ever work on or change the general sexual mindset of the patient. I prefer working with a combination of anatomical information, physical training, and one's own instincts. This should kick-start the sexual system and create new, relaxed desires—and sexual intercourse will eventually usually be possible again.

During the early sessions Katrina was always talking about going clubbing, but gradually this began to tail off. She began to recognize what she had previously been ignoring and to think differently about her nocturnal escapades. She started to feel bad when she fumbled around with others—after all, that meant she was cheating on her husband. Slowly she was taking responsibility for her actions, which resulted in an improved relationship with her husband. She was clearer about what she had in him, but more children? No, thanks! She was certain on that score. After all, they hadn't been having sexual intercourse, although we had an agreed-on goal: penetration.

"Did you used to enjoy sleeping with your husband?" I asked.

"If I'm being honest, I never enjoyed sex with him—his way-too-big schlong banged against my cervix!"

I had to smile—she could speak so naturally now about anatomical realities, and her expression of disgust had disappeared without a trace. I recommended that when they had sex, she tie a piece of silk at the base of his penis to lessen the depth of penetration. This measure had proved successful for many women.

At the next session Katrina said that, at last, she had really slept with her husband.

"And what contraceptives did you use?" I asked.

"It was shortly before my period," she explained, "and my husband withdrew at the right moment." This all seemed a bit odd considering her fears of being pregnant again, and I was reminded about something we had discussed during the first session, namely, sterilization. She thought an operation like that would take care of everything.

I would have liked to continue working with Katrina, but she was free of her vaginismus problem—she could have sex again and, as I later learned, soon after the last session she was sterilized.

10

The Four Spheres of Sexuality

I N MUSIC THERE are interval systems; in medicine, cardiovascular systems. There are political systems, social systems, biological systems, and technical systems, and there is even a systems theory. And, of course, there are sexual systems. The sexuality of each and every person follows a certain logic, depending on everything that they have experienced up until then. As a therapist, I need to understand my client's system and its logic. Why does someone come too soon? Why doesn't a woman like her husband's penis, while other women are profoundly fascinated by these swank manifestations of manhood? Why do some people find their genitals disgusting or even completely ignore them? Others love their genitals. Men in particular are often intrigued by the penis—what's behind that?

In the concept that I use, the French Canadian approach sexocorporealism, a person's sexual system is described as having four important components. These are represented by four spheres, which provide an animated entirety that gives my work a clear structure.

1. THE COGNITION SPHERE

What does a person think about sexuality? Are they prejudiced? Are they ashamed? What do they know, or not know?

2. THE COUPLE SPHERE

This is made up of everything that happens between two people. Is there symbiosis? Are they developing intimacy? Do they talk to each other? Are they both able to seduce one another or others? Are they in love? Is the relationship in trouble?

3. THE PERCEPTION SPHERE

What gender does a person identify as? How do they perceive their body? What are their sexual preferences? What exactly arouses them? Do they have fantasies? Do they feel desire? Are there cravings? What characterizes their sexuality?

4. THE PHYSIOLOGICAL SPHERE

This refers to the body itself. Are there relevant medical diagnoses? Drugs? Viagra? Contraceptives? Alcohol? How do they use their bodies when aroused? Do they have good circulation?

These four groups flow and overlap. If something happens in one, it affects others and influences the entire system. You can visualize this model like wind chimes, constantly in motion. Depending on the wind and weather, the spheres circle in their own spaces, are large or small, are colorful or monochrome, and to a greater or lesser degree are filled with acquired skills, or their absence.

The sexual system these components symbolize develop all through life. With all new clients, it's exciting for me (and them) to discover what the spheres already contain and which of them need encouragement. When a client talks, I listen for components of the four spheres. They specify the structure I use to sort answers and information or, as the case may be, to pose the next question.

Sphere to Sphere

THE LARGEST SEXUAL organ in a human being is ... the brain! This sexual organ is found, logically, in the first area, the Cognition Sphere. It consists of cognitive components like knowledge and ignorance, understanding and preconceptions that people have adopted over the years regarding sexuality—all the things that are externally influenced, such as by sexually charged glossy ads, religious or moral obligations, education, society, or nation. In this way norms develop, as do concepts of what is deviant. These norms and ideas about deviancy could be responsible for a relaxed feeling about nudity (Jennifer) or for qualms about your own body (Katrina or Andrea). Ricarda's story belongs here, as she was also given a very precise and constricted concept of the world and of how men and women interact.

The Cognition Sphere, of course, also has room for the widespread belief that one is not good enough, which is often connected to feelings of extreme shame. Mostly this belief is a relic of childhood, when kids were punished for behavioral "infringements" that were perfectly natural for kids, such as dancing naked in front of a mirror.

The Cognition Sphere is also full of convictions, value judgments, mindsets, and ideals that influence our relationships and sex lives. The "blind spot" that I have referred to a few times also lurks here.

Some examples of worldly wisdom from the Cognition Sphere:

"A gentleman never tells."

"Men are interested in only one thing."

"Blondes are good in bed."

"Redheads are wild."

"Decent girls save themselves."

"We don't talk about that."

"No sex before marriage."

I have a very definite opinion about the last saying. In my kitchen, next to the door to the balcony, a postcard covers a small bump on the wall. Written on it: "No marriage before sex!"

In sex therapy, it's important to scrutinize and reassess counterproductivity or negativity in the Cognition Sphere. New insights open the door to the possibility of new sexual experiences ... and also to love, which leads us directly to the next group.

The Couple Sphere, the second area, is all about relationships, about everything that happens when a partner is nearby. It has to do with being able to have intimate relationships, enjoy the feeling of love, seduction, and communication, but also be competent erotically, which is maybe not so obvious at first. But everybody needs a certain amount of erotic competence. A lot of clients tell me that they feel sexually insecure with their partners, even if they have been together for a long time. They lack erotic experience and confidence in their own capabilities. This includes the competence to recognize their own needs and to communicate them adequately, to be comfortable about presenting themselves sexually, or simply feeling okay about sex. People who prefer sex in the dark know exactly what I mean. The decisive factor is getting used to seeing yourself as a sexual being and finding this fun and pleasurable.

In the Physiological Sphere, various kinds of contact are relevant: stroking, massaging, or pressing the whole body against the partner, caressing, kissing, licking, blowing... Depending on when which technique is used, different stages of arousal will be reached.

Love itself? Yes, when it exists, that too belongs to this sphere because it is directly triggered by neurotransmitters, although being a feeling it also belongs in the next sphere—the Perception Sphere. As a sexologist, however, I often set other priorities. I am primarily concerned with sex—how to improve the quality of sex. To love or not to love? As you like it.

Sometimes treating a sexual theme from the angle of love can even be a hindrance. An example: Women often suffer from lack of orgasms. They talk about their troubles with their gynecologist, where they are often told, "Might there be some sort of tension between you and your husband? Are you having problems letting go?" Such remarks place couples and love at the center of things. They don't consider that the problem might be more to do with the body and sexual technique, which is often the case. Once sexual problems are completely detached from the concept of love, many can be treated.

When I consider the lack of women's orgasms from the perspective of the Cognition Sphere or Physiological Sphere, I often realize that there was a lack of knowledge or that a seemingly obvious opportunity hadn't been taken. On the other hand, with couples, I am inevitably working with *two* individual sexual systems that interact and meet up in the Couple Sphere. They touch each other, and in the best cases, dovetail with other spheres. When couples are sitting with me, I can literally see in front of me what "happens" in this sphere.

Some systems are virtually incompatible: one partner doesn't like the kind of sex that the other does. A prime example of this is fetishes. It is not unusual for both men and women to try early in a relationship to impress their partner by not being entirely truthful about their desires. Sometimes people "forget" to mention their dilemma of choosing leather or whips. Harmonizing two sexual systems can sometimes be a challenge.

The third area, the Perception Sphere, is all about personal sexual preferences—one's own desires and arousals. What do I like? What turns me on? What I consciously think about or what I do with my partner during sex is one thing; the other is what *really* turns me on. That the genitals are aroused (Physiological Sphere) doesn't really tell me always whether a client actually is *feeling* aroused. With men there is a high correlation between actual physical arousal (erection) and the relevant feeling— around 50 percent. With women it's only 10 percent. The penis is like a barometer from which you (and the owner!) can read a man's physical state. The advantage for men is that once the effects of the excitement can be directly verified, it's easier to set up the sexual channels in the brain.

Sexual desires also belong in the Perception Sphere. What's behind these desires? What do I want to do? What am I desiring? Desire is targeted lust.

Sexual fantasies are placed here too. What exactly does the client find arousing? What is the client's role in their fantasies? Are they active or passive, onlookers or participants? As does almost everyone, Chris the fitness freak had little movies in his head that mirrored his sexual system. Both Chris's fantasies and his reality with Elizabeth were about anything but penetration, which, in Chris's case, reflected his troubles with erections.

The last component of this sphere is sexual self-assurance. Is someone happy as a man or woman? What components are to be found in their self-image? Does somebody feel good or bad when compared to others? Gender identity is also important. How does someone feel in their skin? Do they feel they should have been born a different sex?

The fourth group, the Physiological Sphere, is where biological sex is to be found. Is the outward physical appearance of a person male, female, or somewhere in between? Here we are talking about the sex you are born with, not the gender you identify as. Arousal reflexes such as smell, taste, sight, hearing, and touch also belong here. Yet it is not only the sources of our arousal that are significant but also how we use our bodies to create arousal in the first place. What do we do with our body when making love? Are we moving? Quickly or slowly? Are we straining? How are we breathing? What are our hands doing? Our mouths? How can I send my pleasure sky high? Everyone can profit from knowing more about their own and their partners' bodies.

Of course, orgasm also belongs here! It takes many women a long time to learn how to trigger an orgasm because they hardly know anything about their bodies, particularly their genitals, they haven't experimented enough, or they've used inappropriate techniques for arousal. Many women, for instance, increase arousal solely by using pressure. This is sometimes called the *archaic* arousal mode, as it is observed in babies (stimulating themselves through muscle tension and the pressure from their diapers). Some adult women, when masturbating, lie on their stomachs with their legs crossed and press a fist against the clitoris, without even rubbing. With the *mechanical* arousal mode, however, people are aroused mainly through rubbing motions, again with a little pressure and some movement. Additionally, there is an *undulating* arousal mode, which involves moving in all directions with a snakelike action, like a temple dancer, frequently with little muscular tension. Women using this method often say that they seldom achieve an orgasm even though they are very highly aroused. They lack the archaic movements most often needed for orgasms. Finally, the *wave* arousal method, involving the double swing of shoulders, breast area, and pelvis, which provides interplay between muscular tension and relaxation. This sounds a bit funny, doesn't it? I promise you it is! I will describe it later in more detail. These different ways of arousing ourselves are not in series but are parallel to one another, and are often associated with each other.

Medical factors also belong in the Physiological Sphere. Illnesses, for example, that limit the practice or experience of sex, or drugs that people have to take, can also influence arousal or sexual desire. This applies to older clients in particular.

How do the spheres work in practice? A short example.

John was in his mid-forties when he came alone to my office. His problem was erectile dysfunction. He talked about his relationship, explained that he and his wife often argued. In my notebook I wrote down, "Communication," which is a component of the Couple Sphere. He went on to tell me that his parents had not tolerated quarrels, and that they sometimes beat the children when things got out of hand. Here something was happening in the Cognition Sphere, because John had formed very precise views on the subject of what "arguing" meant and linked it to decidedly negative consequences.

Next he said that after one fight, he couldn't sleep with his wife—he didn't feel like it. This, then, was tending toward the Perception Sphere. Many men are affected by unknowns causing erection problems, almost as if the penis itself is at a loss to explain things. They try desperately with rubbing and stroking, but the penis remains limp.

I could try to draw a fairly good picture from all available contexts, could actively look inside each of the spheres and find the right questions. Sometimes I have to work in all four spheres at once. In John's case, however, I asked his wife to join us, so that I could understand the couple's relationship system—after all, the bickering would have to stop. Only after that, I decided, could we get down to solving John's erection problem, should it even still exist.

If the negative associations triggered by a quarrel were the main cause of his tenseness (and thus the erectile dysfunction), then as soon as the couple stopped arguing or argued differently, tension would ease. The vicious circle would be broken—John would then "feel like it" and would probably find it a lot easier to get a hard-on. If, however, over the years he had become accustomed to his arousal methods, during which he hardly breathed or moved, and had already reached a certain age, then his erection troubles would probably persist in some form. It's not only washing machines, fan belts, and jeans that wear out with age. Erections too are no longer as sturdy as they used to be. Therapy would then be directed at improving John's general physical sexual arousal mechanisms (Physiological Sphere). This in turn would affect his mood (Perception and Cognition Spheres), thus establishing a virtuous circle that would support his sense of well-being and relaxation.

I have presented this tour of the spheres in a decidedly simplified form, and first impressions are only suppositions, but it does illustrate the principle. The point is that at any given moment, I know by my client's questions and answers which of the spheres that person is located in and can easily recognize where it is worth delving deeper. And I know when the sphere suddenly changes, when certain issues are being avoided or evaded, which is quite common.

Once I have gauged the logic of the client's sexual system, I can explain the contexts, and clients become more informed about themselves and their situation. Then expanding their potential comes to the foreground. This is now about change, and we embark on the therapy proper.

Out with the Penises!

"YOU'RE BACK AGAIN!" I exclaim as Andrea and I flop into our armchairs. It's one of those rare occasions when I have actually prepared coffee, and it's steaming in our colorful mugs.

"Out with the penises!" I say after we've had a sip. The brown paper bag with the silicon penises lies ready on the small Danish table next to my chair. I pick it up and rustle it a little, which results in Andrea sitting there not quite as relaxed as she was at the beginning. I then fish a medium-sized penis out of the bag and lean slightly forward.

"The Floppy Horror Penis Show!" I whisper with an enticing expression and throw the penis to her. Bull's-eye! She catches it. "Eeeeee!" That little screech is precisely the reason that I wanted to work in her Physiological Sphere for this session. It should then be able to influence her Perception and Cognition Spheres.

"Do you like it?" I ask with a serious expression.

"Somehow not really...Although...Actually, it *does* feel pretty cuddly."

"Hmm." I wait while she fumbles around with the penis.

"I often worry that I don't really touch Harold the right way," she said after a while.

I decide to teach Andrea the anatomy of the penis, making her aware of the testicles, which a great many women ignore while having sex (far too sensitive, they think). But many men enjoy being touched, kissed, and licked there (and further along). And how! Andrea is surprised to hear this and starts asking questions: "Where's the penis most sensitive? Is it the same for all men?" While I answer one question after the other and explain even more, Andrea gradually becomes less shy. She now holds the soft silicon penis calmly.

I remember her homework from the last session: to have "a good look down below" at her own genitals. I had also suggested that after having had a good look at the outside, she could try exploring inside with her own fingers. She said, however, that she would prefer to use a dildo if things got that far but she didn't have one, which is why I said that she could use an ordinary carrot, slipping a condom I'd already given her over it. But—and most importantly—I insisted that she continue with her "down below" exercises only when the time and place were right (warm room, soft music, just after a warm bath . . . and no children nearby).

To nudge Andrea in the right direction, I ask her how it feels when Harold touches her.

"There's a pulsating feeling at the opening, on the lips. And when he goes deeper with his fingers, it feels like I have to pee."

Many women say this, because there is a prostate-like tissue right at the entrance to the vagina, only about an inch in. This tissue has many glands and canals that surround the urethra and the urethral opening leading to the mucous membrane. When there's slight finger pressure on this tissue, the brain links it to the need to pee, not to sexual desire. Sexual desire comes into play only when the original response (peeing) is pushed to the background by the sexual drive, and this requires sexual synaptic links in the brain.

"Andrea, you seem to like it when Harold touches you, am I right?"

"Yes."

"What happens next?"

"He strokes my vagina and—"

"Sorry to interrupt you, but do you really mean vagina? I think you mean on the outside—the vulva."

"Oh, yes! I forgot!" She then continues her account: "My legs are stretched and crossed, then there's shivering and twitching and I have to stop. I'm sure there's more to come, but then I would have to uncross my legs . . ."

"Is the shivering and twitching pleasant?"

"I guess so, especially when it starts. And when Harold puts his fingers inside me, that's great. But afterward I squeeze my legs together even tighter, and suddenly it begins to hurt, as if it's too narrow. My gynecologist says that's normal for women my age."

Andrea is beginning to speak freely and I'm very pleased about that, but I have to intervene. If as a therapist I don't correct misleading information, it becomes hard fact.

"Just a moment! That bit about becoming narrow with age is one of the many myths that circulate about our sex. It's not strictly true. The vagina does lose some elastic tissues over the years and if it isn't stretched now and then, it can actually shrink a bit. So if a woman doesn't have sex for years, it *is* possible for the passage to become so narrow that you can only enter it with your finger. But as long as a woman has sex occasionally, this doesn't apply."

Andrea looks at me skeptically—her gynecologist had suggested the opposite.

I continue. "For women going through menopause or just past it who've been single for a while, I recommend playing with the vagina a bit before having sex again, just to get it used to having visitors. But you aren't nearly that old." I look at Andrea to see her reaction: it's important for her to understand. "I think this feeling of tightness comes from you bracing yourself."

"That may well be true," she concedes.

"It seems to me that you're good at being aware—you tense yourself and you feel the tightness. So what are we going to do about it?"

"I'll have to stop tensing myself?"

"Nobody *has* to do *anything* here, ever. But what we could do now to begin with is a little exercise using your fist as a model for your vulva and vagina." I show Andrea my loosely clenched fist and ask her to clench hers the same way.

I use this exercise with many clients to simulate the vulva and, later, penetration. We look at the thumb side of the fist. The upper joint of the index finger represents the clitoris. The curled-up index finger tucked into the base of the thumb forms the entrance to the vulva. (Go on, try it!) With the aid of this model, a woman can explain to me pretty precisely how she touches and strokes herself (I usually go through the actions myself, using my hands). She can also enter this "snail" with a finger from the other hand.

The idea is for Andrea to discover the different sensations, just as it was for Katrina with the fleshlight: first to try to slip into the soft, loosely clenched fist, then to try the same with a tightly clenched fist. After that I fetch a lube tube, smear lube onto the fist and fingers, and repeat the exercise. The tighter Andrea clenches her fist, the more difficult it is for her to slide her finger in—even the gel makes little difference.

Andrea is putting a lot of effort just into clenching her fist.

"See how your fist is almost drained of blood when you do that?" She nods. "The natural moistness of arousal happens because tiny vessels in the lower tissues of the vagina that are well supplied with blood expand and release moisture." I let my explanation sink in for a few moments and, while she looks at her anemic fist, slowly the penny drops.

"Oh, so no wonder nothing happens when my legs are all tensed up." She looks properly relieved.

"Precisely!"

Andrea opens up her fist and wipes her hands with a tissue, then grabs the silicon penis that was still lying on the sofa next to her and suddenly tells me that she is thinking, before the next session, of trying to have sex with her legs uncrossed, to discover whether the new position makes any difference. I nod.

"I lost my virginity at twenty-one," she continues. "I was looking for any available male. He was twenty-five and looked okay. It didn't hurt—I just didn't get any pleasure out of it. It was a kind of confrontation therapy. I just wanted to get the whole thing behind me." Andrea's eyes light up: thinking back to a time when she had control over her actions seems to have given her positive energy.

I try digging a little deeper. "What do you mean by 'confrontation therapy'?" The phrase came across very hard and direct, almost as if she was spitting it out.

Andrea tilts her head. "My friends had all already had sex for the first time. I was the only one scared of it. I hoped that after that, I would like sex, but it wasn't to be."

"It sounds like your approach was both a good and a bad idea."

"It was okay. But I didn't suddenly feel like a woman after, like I was expecting to. I still felt like a kid."

"What was it like for you when your breasts started to develop? That's something very female, isn't it?" Andrea has told me a number of times that she doesn't like her body.

"I liked them a lot." She beams. "But I didn't allow myself this feeling."

Finally, she's in the Perception Sphere. She tells me that she hated it when her father, with a dirty grin, grabbed her mother's breasts in front of her. Her mother would retaliate by grabbing her husband in the crotch and saying, "Well, how do *you* like it?"

Andrea's father once said to her, "Lovely dress, sweetheart, but didn't they have one in your size?"

I'm not surprised after that when Andrea tells me she dressed in shapeless clothing during puberty so that nobody could see the new shape of her womanhood—many girls do this.

She says, "My father was the bad guy and my mother was the victim."

This makes me think. Many clients talk at first about a problem parent and continue to focus on this parent, only to later reveal that the real problem is the other parent. With Andrea it was her father: in her opinion, he behaved in a way that was anything but affectionate. But in the course of therapy, as the image of her mother gradually takes shape, the real picture emerges. Although Andrea tries to convince me that her mother was a victim, she was most definitely not. Grabbing someone in the crotch and making snide remarks as retaliation for being mistreated are not acts typical of victims. And the following story too: Andrea locked herself in her room after a quarrel with her mother, but with velvety words, her mother eventually persuaded her to open the door, and then when Andrea did, she beat her.

"It only happened once," says Andrea, apologizing for her mother. Time and again it's the same mechanisms that grind into action: symbiotic children (now grown up) can hardly bear directing blame where it belongs—on the parents.

"Does it need to be more than once to be considered deliberate and bad?" I ask. "Did your mother realize how you would feel being cheated like that?"

Andrea nods.

Her mother wasn't a victim. Rather, she behaved like an offender. This reminds Andrea of something else. During a family holiday when Andrea was seventeen, her mother, hiding in the bushes, watched her daughter kiss and cuddle someone else, and later confronted her about every detail—not particularly promising for a girl on the verge of adulthood. Since then Andrea has had to live with the thought that her mother caught her in her early attempts at petting and continued to spy. I can see how these thoughts still plague her—hardly surprising as her mother crossed a boundary and gate-crashed her daughter's sexuality.

"Children are worthless. Adults always win." This, in a nutshell, is how Andrea describes her childhood experiences.

I let these thoughts stand and go back to my original remark.

"Do you feel your body tensing when you talk about your mother?"

She nods, while still playing with the penis. She doesn't seem to notice she's doing it.

"Have you tried out the carrot yet?"

Although it's a big jump, I want to get back to the actual issue—the female anatomy. I think that Andrea's inner turmoil might actually help get things moving and bring about change. She has opened up now, as if she knows my intentions, she looks at me almost defiantly, but then she lets her defenses down. It's too late for secrets.

"It was pretty cold ... and it hurt a bit ... ," she says.

"What do you mean, 'cold'?"

To begin with, she says, she dodged putting the carrot inside her. Then last weekend she decided to take action (she felt good about that). She quickly fetched the carrot out of the fridge and, without a condom, pushed it into her vagina. She briefly asked herself if the carrot wasn't too cold, but dropped the thought.

"I didn't really want to do it." She looks at me as if to say that she thinks the whole exercise was nuts.

"Why not?"

"Because it was cold . . . It almost hurt."

"You don't say!" I can't help bursting out laughing. And Andrea joins me. It's equally liberating and absurd. But how little some women value their sexual organs! If she had had a positive, favorable feeling toward her female anatomy, she wouldn't have deep-frozen it with an ice-cold carrot.

I use her "cool" experience to try to emphasize how insensitively she has acted toward her body up till now. She almost has a guilty conscience about the whole affair now, which I think is thoroughly appropriate. Why did she put a cold carrot inside her when her instincts were telling her that it wasn't a good idea? It slowly dawns on me that she has got used to brushing aside her own feelings— simply ignoring them—but that she generally felt good about them. She thought about parboiling the carrot before the next attempt and putting it in while it's lukewarm.

"Hmmm," she adds. "Roasted parsnips!"

I laugh and wonder if the next attempt will involve possible scalding.

I notice how the whole time she's been talking she has continued to pet and prod the flesh-colored penis. For almost twenty minutes she's bent it back and forth cautiously, stroking and holding it, almost as if it's a comfort object.

Suddenly she realizes this. "Oh, here I am sitting with a penis in my hands the whole time!" An expression of astonishment and enjoyment crosses her face.

"Yes, and I didn't want to disturb you," I say happily. Then, on the spur of the moment, I take one of the other penises out of the bag and place it on my crotch (as always, I'm wearing jeans). I've never done anything like this before. It feels really good to see "my own" penis lying there, to touch it, move it to the side, or just hold it. I draw Andrea's attention to "my" penis. It's a pleasurable feeling, and all of a sudden I can imagine why this dangly thing is so important to most men. Andrea feels just the same, and there we sit with our great, limp penises in our laps.

"Can you imagine being able to treat your own body like this?" I ask. "And your husband's penis?"

"Of course!"

I have the impression that she's telling the truth, as it's extremely difficult to separate Andrea from her penis.

"I'm ready," she says and ends the session.

Three weeks later I get an email from Andrea:

Dear Ann-Marlene!

I just have to tell you how I've been getting on. I was, after my (ice cold!) experience, not really keen on shoving something in down below again. But on Friday evening when Harold was taking the kids swimming, I spontaneously decided: what the heck—now or never. It can't go on like this! Cue the carrot. Somehow I was really hot (the carrot was lukewarm!), and I tried it. It was funny feeling myself. But I kept going and what can I say—I was faithful to the carrot during the next few days. (I don't always just make a pot of tea now when Harold goes out in the evening with the dog!) And now? It works! It is IN-CREDIBLE! I can have orgasms. And not just one!

A well-stirred (not shaken) cocktail made of curiosity, courage, endurance, and relaxation can sometimes work miracles. Andrea has just discovered her favorite drink, and will soon be taking Harold on a date without the ice. Although—ice used in the right places...

The Trailblazers

MANY SEX RESEARCHERS and educators have enabled me to practice therapy the way I do. The pioneers were, among others, the Scotswoman Marie Stopes, whose book, *Married Love or Love in Marriage,* published in 1918, was initially refused by publishers because her subject matter was considered too hot to handle. Stopes wrote about sex and the link between ovulation and sexual desire.

The Kinsey Institute I've already mentioned. Alfred Charles Kinsey was actually a professor of zoology—an entomologist. At some point he was assigned to be a student marriage counselor, a job he became so interested in that he soon began to study people and their sexuality. He carried out the first empirical studies on sexuality and thus laid the foundations for scientific sexual research. He devised the first questionnaires and observed, from behind a hidden screen, exactly what was happening physiologically during the act of sex. Prostitutes who he had hired had sex with male test subjects. He was fiercely criticized and discredited for this, but to this day his studies haven't lost any validity among sexologists.

In the 1970s the sex researchers Virginia Johnson and William Masters followed in Kinsey's footsteps. Over the course of many years they studied sex even more precisely than the former bug man. Thousands of volunteers were wired with electrodes under laboratory conditions to reveal the procession of events that happen during the sex act.

Masters and Johnson designed much of the equipment they needed themselves. On the basis of their studies, they formulated their now famous human sexual response cycle.

All sex researchers describe models of sexual systems that are shaped by their respective social and scientific perceptions. Over the decades these have become ever more complete and comprehensive. Now we see things more from a neurological perspective—only once there are changes inside the head can sex therapy be a success.

11

Come On!

MEN AND THEIR BODIES

Ms. Henning!
Did you know that the length of cohabitation can be expo-
nentially graded by modulation of the state of arousal of the
penis? With sequentially high frictional frequency and the
subsequent retardation of frequency, respectively, conjuga-
tion remains initially without ejaculation!
Yours, B.

You have already read a number of emails to me, but this one I would like to translate for you: "If you vary the tempo of thrusts, you can regulate arousal and thus extend the time of sexual intercourse!"

And that's exactly what we're just about to tackle.

Let me introduce Alan (35), Roland (46), Arnold (65), and Simon (24)—four men I've worked with (mainly within the Physiological Sphere) and with whom I had a certain amount of success.

The One Who Came Too Soon

IT WAS PITCH black outside when Alan came for his 7:00 a.m. winter appointments, punctual to the minute. A lawyer, he had to be in his office by nine. Alan worked in the law firm of his future (hopefully) father-in-law, the idea being that at some stage later he would run the firm. For every appointment, he chose the same place to sit, on the red sofa. His suit was always immaculate, and to complete the picture of his perfect styling, he chose white shirts and unobtrusively striped ties. He looked good, particularly as his dark curly hair didn't seem to always want follow the rules of etiquette despite attempts to control it with copious amounts of gel. Troublemaker!

Even his briefcase had its special place—at his feet on the cognac-colored parquet floor, covering a scorch mark. Someone must have stubbed out a cigarette there before I took over the office. I filed the mark under "That's life," but my impression was that Alan wasn't fond of blemishes. It seemed as if it *had* to be removed, as if it didn't fit in with his idea of an orderly world.

Analogous to Alan's early appointment was his problem: coming too soon during intercourse, a.k.a. premature ejaculation (PE). He had been together with his thirty-two-year-old girlfriend, Jacqueline, for only a year and a half. She had accompanied him to one session—a self-confident redhead with green eyes and freckles who seemed to have her life well under control. She worked as a film editor and, as she put it, wanted plenty and extensive sex.

"Coming too soon"—this expression covers quite a range. Coming too soon can mean that someone only just manages to penetrate before coming, but it can also mean having an orgasm after a few thrusts; sometimes even a couple of minutes of sex is possible. Of course there's a concrete medical definition for PE. It doesn't count the minutes or the number of thrusts—merely states that a man is not in the position to extend the moment of ejaculation during intercourse: he comes too early for what he or his partner would consider to be satisfactory sex.

I have my own, slightly modified, definition of PE: A client suffers from it when he is unable to have the protracted sex he would like to have. I see the whole thing as very subjective. And just another interesting thought: in the course of evolution, the ones who came too soon were probably the superheroes. They survived because they *weren't* marathon screwers, who were more likely to be set upon by their enemies. After all, as far as procreation is concerned, all you need to do is unload the seeds—extended pleasure is immaterial.

Alan explained: "Sometimes even on the way into the vagina, I'm already having an orgasm. Only on good days can I hold out for up to a minute." He was sad about it, and also disappointed that in many situations his premature ejaculation had limited enjoyment for both him and his girlfriend, and still often did. "The typical weekend where breakfast in bed is followed by hours of sex was never really an option for me." Although not many emotions were shown in his face, I still felt that there was a great romantic longing in him.

"Is it different when you masturbate?" I asked.

Alan's eyes brightened. "Yes, and with blow jobs. And if sex is spontaneous. Then I just don't have time to think about things." Up until then, Alan had told all his partners right at the start of their relationship that he came early, in the hope that his tension would decrease and he could hold out a little longer. That wasn't the case, and this strategy had never worked for him.

Alan's account is prime example of a vicious circle: the client thinks he knows what will happen, and is scared. Expecting this unhappy outcome, he becomes tense, and exactly what he was trying to avoid happens: he comes. But even worse, his fears have been confirmed, and next time he will be just as worried, if not more so.

With every kind of anxiety—including the fear of coming too soon—the brain's warning system is alerted. The three options of handling potential dangers are activated: escape, attack, or freeze. Whichever path is chosen, more subconsciously than consciously, one thing is clear: this is definitely *not* the right time for pleasure and relaxation! The amygdala sounds the alarm and the pelvic floor muscles contract and any thoughts of erections have to be dampened as quickly as possible. This means "Discharge! At once!" My assistant, Anika, once said, "I guess it's hard to run away when you've got a boner!"

I wanted to know from Alan when this tension and fear were strongest. Before I could ask him, however, he said, "Some positions are better than others. I have more time for thrusting if we're spooning. I've also tried distracting myself by thinking about boring people or counting backward— like counting sheep if you can't sleep, but the other way around. Neither helped."

I can well believe that. The problem for many men who come too soon lies precisely in their attention *not* being on their penises. If they count or think about boring things, they're trying to lessen their excitation. But to buck this, the attention must be *on* the penis. Otherwise, the counting becomes a countdown to just that—ejaculation!

By using diagrams, I explain to Alan how tension affects his lower body. A simple drawing of a man with a round belly, a bum, and a penis demonstrates how a proper pressure chamber comes into existence: the diaphragm being the lid, and the pelvic floor running all the way around to the behind, the boiler. Everything contracts. In the boiler the pressure continues to increase. The upper thighs, shoulders, and neck (well, actually, all the large muscle groups) help out by creating more tension in the body until it begins to bubble in the "boiler" and the man comes. People who want to reproduce this phenomenon? Firmly clench both your fists—your arm muscles also become tense. It takes just a few seconds for the brain to broadcast the command: "Okay! Let go!"

Alan described his problem discerningly. Without knowing the interrelationships, he still managed to figure out quite a lot. I had already had other clients use his strategies for solving their problem (distracting themselves and counting backward), but these have never proved adequate for coping with PE. The important key words, however, had at long last been raised: *muscle tension.*

Men generally have higher muscle tone than women. Additional tension comes from stressful routines. "Just grit your teeth!" the men say, or, "Pull yourself together!" If the jaw is tense, as I have already said, tension is triggered in the pelvic floor too. It's just that most people don't realize it. Still we sit in front of our computers for hours on end, making ourselves tense and stiff. In a body that is always tense, arousal is unlikely to spread even during sex. This fits with what Alan said about his climaxes being generally short: "Only sometimes, when foreplay is longer, are orgasms fantastic."

Alan came for therapy for five months, and we often worked physically (dressed and without touching). For many clients, this is all about feeling and getting in touch with their own bodies, and not only sexually. A more precise and finely tuned awareness can be learned. Alan also needed to pay more attention to his penis at home, to place his hand on it, whether in the shower or in bed. When masturbating, he needed to learn to play with his arousal to find out what it feels like, maybe find variations in his penis's sensitivity. He needed just to try to get to know his pride and joy a little better.

I also wanted to solve the problem of his distinctive jaw tenseness. We began by getting him to move his jaw in all directions. With his mouth wide open, Alan yawned and stuck his tongue out. I also asked him to note how tense his jaw was during sex. He knew immediately what I meant: "I tense *everything,* even when I masturbate. I press my tongue against my gums, clench my teeth, and can hardly breathe. My balls really rise—it's a very secure grip." Later, when I asked his girlfriend, Jacqueline, about it, she nodded and said that he "worked hard" during sex. His whole face would become distorted. You couldn't put it clearer than that.

A little later, when Alan told me he didn't really want to think about the tension in his jaw and pelvic floor during sex, I suggested that he try chewing gum, as the motion relaxes the jaw. At some stage the new behavior would become normal and he could drop using the chewing gum during intercourse. He liked the idea. Jacqueline was willing to try anything to solve the problem. Both of them approached it pragmatically and laughed a lot in the process. Laughter not only raises the spirits, it's good for the pelvic floor too.

The work with Alan's body continued. I rolled out the red yoga mat that Alan would use for his exercises to get used to feeling himself more intensively. The idea was for him to firmly tense all the muscles of his limbs individually, one after the other, from the soles of his feet to the neck and head, and then to relax them. Later we stood in front of the full-sized mirror to mobilize the pelvis, get it moving. Doing this in front of a mirror helps to achieve a perfect linkage between muscular tension, tempo, and movement. The client stands there, feet a bit apart, with slightly bent knees, looking a bit like an ape. The center of gravity is slightly forward, roughly in line with the toes. In this position the pelvis is free to be moved forward or backward and to swing—and with it the wonderful bulge in the pants. Highly erotic!

However, the upper thighs and pelvis often move more like a rigid unit, especially when the man moves only his knees up and down. The pelvis itself then remains almost immobile. Bending your knees doesn't sound quite as relaxing as swinging your hips, though, does it? With Alan, however, everything was fine: his pelvis became increasingly loose, in a positive sense.

It's generally thought to be inappropriate for men and women swing into action with their pelvises. Sexologists, however, see it as essential.

"Don't be surprised if something gets excited—that's what it's all about," I sometimes say to my clients during these exercises. If the men are doing it right, they instantly feel the difference. A bit of self-consciousness is allowed. After all, they're watching their own manhood gyrate or thrust, and that in the presence of their female therapist! In a couple of cases, men have all of a sudden had to go home early. To practice, of course!

Alan, incidentally, enjoyed the exercises, pelvic movements being lewd or not. His sense of suffering was high, so he was motivated. He knew that Jacqueline wanted to feel him inside her for more than two or three thrusts. He was worried that she might leave him if he couldn't get the problem under control.

From his perspective, it was all his fault. Sex therapists, however, consider coming too soon generally to be a couples' problem. Although it's the man's role to learn to control his arousal, how the partner copes with PE is just as important. Jacqueline could have been unintentionally exerting pressure, maybe because she was frustrated at always having to halt her sexual desires when he accidentally came. There had to be room for and understanding of her needs too. PE has a great influence on sex—for both parties.

The poster for the 1990s German comedy released in English as *Maybe . . . Maybe Not* was a cartoon figure of a naked man who had somehow got himself tied in a knot. In the practice of sexology, we "unknot" people both physiologically and psychologically. Fundamentally, Alan had an upright, centralized, straight posture, but he kept his upper body as taut as an umbrella. In Denmark we call such people *Knudemanden*, which means something like "knot men."

There was hardly any movement in Alan's chest area, and he also had hardly any facial expression. This for me was an indication that I should soon set up a "movement upstairs" program. The objective of this program is to get the client moving both emotionally and physically. The first movement we practice affects the shoulders, chest, neck, and head. How does it work? To begin, we lean slightly forward, as if we're about to gently pick up a baby. The countermovement involves straightening up with the arms stretched slightly behind so that the chest projects (without a baby).

Alan had already mastered the pelvic exercises we had practiced in front of the mirror. This we then incorporated in with the new chest movements in such a way that the whole body was in motion. The idea was that from then on, Alan should be able to control his passions by playing with muscular tension, tempo, and the dimensions of his movements.

Physically, full-body movement puts into effect completely natural processes, just like coughing or laughing: the pelvis projects, shoulders become rounded, and the chin rises slightly. We exhale. Afterward the pelvis retreats, shoulders drop, the chest swells to take in air. You're welcome to try it. You can do it sitting or lying—indeed, you can carry out the movements in any position, including, later, during sex. You can picture it like this: After a hunched back comes a hollow back, and again a hunched back, which becomes a hollow back, and so on. All this is very good for the circulation, and the brain receives more information during sex. Feeling more means more passion.

I also suggested that Alan used a fleshlight for further home exercises. You remember the silicon vagina men can practice their thrusts with? When using a fleshlight, it is not moved back and forth (like the hand when masturbating). Instead, men use it as a training device, thrusting into it from the pelvis. Whether fast or slow, deep or shallow, relaxed or tense would be for Alan to find out. All in good time.

The interesting and wonderful thing is that the physical exercises we practice also initiate psychological stability. Sometimes we forget that the things that we physically do influence our thoughts. And that is exactly the point of these exercises—the new bodily flexibility should have a positive impact on emotions and performance. Later, men can manage their masculinity more consciously. They can stand up for their opinions and seduce their partners with more confidence, regardless of whether they're on a sexual adventure or in a long-term relationship. They are hungry and want something, and for this they are now able to rely on their bodies.

Many men, especially of Alan's generation, want to "do the right thing" for women, not just in a sexual context, and sometimes to the extent of ignoring their own needs. Their independent partners, however, don't hide their erotic desires and need someone who can generally stand their ground—not only but also in bed.

At the beginning of his therapy, Alan was so fixated on Jacqueline's needs that he was always tense in her presence and wanted to do everything right. He told me that compared to her, he felt inadequate and insecure. Why was that?

Alan's father disappeared from the scene early in Alan's childhood, and he grew up as the youngest child with his mother and four sisters. He was surrounded by older and thus stronger women, and compared to them he felt small. This, evidently, would come back to plague him in his love life: in his private life he could hardly ever speak his mind to women—in his job, that was a different matter.

There is a sexocorporeal model that describes the path to manhood every boy takes. It's a circle split into two halves by a vertical line. The two halves are joined by an elongated bridge. On the left are women; on the right, men.

Although born to the mother and symbiotically linked to her, a boy soon discovers that his body and hers are different. Those like him—the men—he has yet to find. The process causes fear as the young man has to leave the security of the nest and mother and "cross the bridge" to reach the men's camp. He might not arrive unharmed: on the way he doesn't meet only positive role models but sometimes the opposite. Of course many men take a pleasant stroll across the metaphorical bridge, looking back happily at the women. We sexologists then say they're "well anchored to their masculinity." Such men, in our model, are linked in a relaxed way to their gender and their roles as men. They are free of—and for—women.

The model of the divided circle can also theoretically describe two other types of men: those with an unbalanced relationship to women and those with an unbalanced relationship to their own sex. The one group is drawn to strong women. They ally themselves with women, adulate them, and keep their opinions to themselves. In short, they more or less forfeit their own needs for women's. Back in our circle, the dividing line between the genders in this model is now so far to the right that the men are squeezed together while the women take up most of the space.

In the opposite group is the macho man. He is in no way allied to women but tries to repress them in order to exaggerate his own insecure manliness. Macho men say, "Only a man can understand." Or, "This is no place for a woman." Macho men move the dividing line so far to the left that there is hardly room for women. In the stereotype of this model, it is the women who get the raw deal, in part because they don't rebel against the control the men have. Both extremes, the woman-lover (termed heterocentrically, as he focuses on his female counterpart) and the macho man (egocentric, as he himself is the pivot in his world) are not at ease with their masculinity, which often has an influence on erections.

Figuratively, for a "soft" man the penis is hanging limply in the women's camp—at least it feels like that to him, since, psychologically, the stronger woman has emasculated him. The macho man's penis is proud and erect, be it in his mind, by means of Viagra, or through a penis substitute like a sports car or pumped-up muscles. Often younger, showy women give him a feeling of potency. He needs this, as unfortunately, in real life, his pride and joy is not particularly reliable. In principle, I don't have anything against Viagra, Porsches, muscles, or sex bombs; I just want to say that these things all have a soothing effect on our macho man because they help him to externally project the image of the prize stud that, internally, he certainly is not.

Heterocentric Alan gradually began to speak his mind in front of Jacqueline and to stand up for his opinions. What up until then was linked to the risk of being rejected by his partner he now slowly found to come naturally, without being macho. He was no longer willing to be bossed around by Jacqueline. At first they quarreled more, but soon his fears diminished, which had a positive effect on the relationship because his girlfriend wanted nothing more than an opposite number she could feel was a full partner.

If now and then Alan fell back to his old patterns of muting and holding back, Jacqueline immediately nagged him: there was still work to do, which is why I was all the more surprised to hear Alan tell me that Jacqueline was pregnant and that he had proposed to her. *It's going to be exciting!* I thought. *They'll have their fights, but I'm pretty confident that they'll make it.*

Becoming Slower Quickly

A PHYSIOTHERAPIST I know and value highly, Astrid Land-messer, said to me after a course on the pelvic floor and sexuality, "If only men knew that they could hold back the urge to ejaculate by learning to control parts of the pelvic floor, they'd have a totally different experience of sex." And she was absolutely right! Variation is important—from relaxation to flexible tension. "Like a yo-yo," said Astrid.

Roland was forty-six, a wiry IT engineer with a mountain of hair on his oval head. He had been married for four years. He, like Alan, was suffering from PE. In the end his was a textbook case: attended lessons, understood lessons, did homework, reported back, fine-tuned, problem solved! He came to my practice three times, then everything continued on its own from there.

"God knows I've tried everything, but nothing's worked," he said at the first session. Roland came when he held his penis to guide it into his wife. "Good for contraception," he quipped.

"What else have you noticed?" I asked.

"The second try, after coming, is slightly better. From behind is a total disaster!" Unfortunately, Roland's wife was particularly fond of being taken "really hard" from behind—she associated it with porn-like passion.

Roland explained how even masturbation was mostly hurried—his penis reacted rapidly. "Until I was seventeen, I shared a room with my older brother. A friend of his often spent the night there too. I had to do it quietly." The way he masturbated as a teenager had an effect on his later sexual behavior. Many kids start by exploring privately under the bedsheets, with bated breath. Later, within the confines of their own apartments, they can change their methods of sexual gratification, but most people don't—the old way worked just fine! Until... well, until the old pattern *has* to be changed, out of necessity.

Ronald the Quick, my secret name for him, spoke to his partner openly and calmly about his arousal issues. He told her about the issues we covered in our first session. They tried the less stimulating positions out. Sometimes he lay relaxed on his back with his wife on top of him, and that lasted a bit longer. The next time he stood. Success: he managed two thrusts and straight away he was ready for another try. "On the living room table with a view of her magnificent breasts, I managed to hold on!" In the best of moods, he practiced daily, used and stretched the pelvic-floor muscles that he got to know on the red yoga mat. (It feels a little like peeing when you're in a hurry.) When Roland was just about to ejaculate, he would combine pelvic stretching with deep inhalation, which relaxes the diaphragm, the belly muscles, and the pelvis before the pressure chamber explodes.

Roland trained with the vigor of a professional athlete shortly before a championship game. His thought: *I feel I'm heading in the right direction, so I'll just carry on.* For me as a therapist, that's the sign of a successfully closed case.

On All Fours

ARNOLD WAS A urologist who asked for an appointment after attending one of my lectures. He came to my practice with erectile dysfunction (ED). He couldn't maintain an erection during sexual intercourse. Now he was no longer even able to penetrate his wife, Charlotte (in her mid-forties), and was having more difficulty achieving an orgasm than he used to, which was prompting considerable uncertainty in his wife. She was even doubting whether her husband loved her at all. (Here we go again!)

Even though he was a doctor, the physical connections that happen in sexual arousal were new to the slightly plump Arnold with a bushy mustache. After I had explained most of it, I got him down on all fours on the yoga mat, because in this position the pelvis is relaxed. So there "hung" Arnold, initially with a quizzical expression on his face, swinging his pelvis.

"Pay attention to what you feel," I said.

He continued without anything seeming to happen. But after a while his expression changed. Something was happening... and not to the perfectly pruned mustache! Typical doctor—when physical realities bumped into scientific interest, Harold looked at me and said, "Oh! I *am* feeling something. My penis is getting stiff... Now, that's exciting!" A eureka moment for him!

With this and other exercises, clients begin to understand that they have bodily systems that they can influence. To alter these systems, however, exercises are needed. An instructor once said to me that there are hundreds even sometimes thousands of "channels" to follow before the body internalizes the changes in a certain sexual process. But what are these "channels"? Even when you're brushing your teeth, you can move your pelvis back and forth. When done correctly (and linked to the desired associations), that can certainly count as a "channel"—something is happening. What you do doesn't always have to be complete courses of exercises: it's more about awareness.

Arnold wasn't nearly far enough along this path. His problem was so extreme that he was no longer able to ejaculate. He hadn't had an orgasm for ages. The situation did improve with exercises, though. Once during sex with Charlotte he even almost came, but then, seconds before he was about to reach his climax, she moaned into his ear, "Get on with it!" And with that it was over—Arnold didn't come. So much can be said on the topic of partner pressure! Arnold was sad and distressed about it when he told me, as he hadn't been so close to an orgasm for years. He felt as if he had to start all over again—a pity.

Heartache or High Point?

SIMON, A BUS driver, the last in this group of men, was a pale young man with straight dark hair. His case too shows how easy it can be to make change possible. When he came to the practice, he was suffering from heartache. By then two girlfriends had already given him the shove. The reason was the same in both cases—he came too early.

We arranged two appointments, during which I explained the physiological connections, practiced exercises with him, and gave him some homework. Simon couldn't afford more appointments, but the ones we had proved quite sufficient. A few weeks later he wrote me an email:

> I used the lube you recommended. I've never tried anything like it for masturbating, and it was a very different feeling to give my penis a treat with a wet and slippery hand. I'm also trying to work on my pelvis and on relaxation techniques for my whole body. First I watched your blog videos on thrusting movements—really well made.

*After that I masturbated for about fifteen minutes, with
highs and lows, until I had an orgasm. I could restrain it
as long as I wanted! I also noticed that when I fantasize
and rub intensely, I reach a point of no return, but if I
slow down and try to think of nothing, then the excitation
curve dips. In the end I just wanted an orgasm, and I
think it was totally different from normal. The spurt had a
lot more energy—it really came shooting out. I hope that's
a good sign. I fell asleep with a huge grin on my face, was
over the moon. Now I can hardly wait for my first controlled sex, where I can decide when to come.*

Someone was getting a taste for it! Simon, in his email,
depicted what good self-stimulation is like and how you can
practice and play around with arousal.

A couple of months later I received a final email from
Simon:

*At last I've had my first go at really long sex with a woman
who is experienced and ten years older than me [she was
thirty-four]. It lasted the whole night, and she wants to see
me again.*

It was signed "The Casanova of Reinbek."

12

Macho Men

MANY PEOPLE ASK, "How can I have pleasurable, sensual sex with my long-term partner?" People freshly in love don't have to think about this question much—they sleep with each other whenever and wherever possible and as often as time allows. In the car. In bed. Somewhere out in the open (hopefully, no one's watching!). Sometimes there might be little hints that the new flame's art of seduction leaves something to be desired—a lack of sensitivity, maybe, in a particular technique. But in the freshly-in-love phase, you don't ponder such things long. Mostly, people just get down to business without extended foreplay. After all, you're hot for each other. Hormones go crazy; everything else, you assume, will somehow sort itself out. But unfortunately, it doesn't. In the course of a relationship, the sex repertoire remains much as it was during the phase of first being in love. Someone who tends toward clumsiness will not suddenly become a gentle stroker. And an innocent, sensitive lover will not suddenly turn into a red-hot seducer. (These stereotypes can be found in women as well as men, of course.)

The inevitable finally happens and after the first wild phase, previously suppressed needs begin to surface. He thinks, *Why, oh why, can't she just give me a decent blow job? All this leisurely licking is definitely not turning me on!* This might even lead to doubts: *Was she faking passion early on? Why doesn't she moan softly like she used to?* And maybe she thinks, *Why doesn't he understand how little I like all this nipple-rubbing? Why don't we talk more?*

In this phase of realization, very different questions need to be asked. What does this relationship to this person actually give me? Can I continue to develop through the relationship, and in what way? As a man or woman, what role do I adopt toward this person, and how do I feel about it? Can both sex and love survive?

Sometimes it helps to remember that the elastic-band dynamics of sex and love are not always equally good. There are ups and downs and, above all, things will never be the same as they were at the beginning. Over the course of years, maintaining excitement takes a fair amount of effort, and both partners have to contribute. You have to be prepared for the chance of being wounded. Talking to each other also becomes increasingly important when routines kick in and the brain switches to automatic. Nevertheless, and precisely for this reason, everyone should ask themselves at regular intervals: *How am I really doing with my partner?*

I still remember Nick and Hannah well. He was thirty-seven, and she was a year older. They'd known each other for two years before marrying and now had four children. When they first came to my practice, the youngest child, a girl, was just six months old and was sleeping in her carrier. At that point, Nick and Hannah had been a couple for eight years. They could in no way be compared to Harold and

Andrea—not the slightest hint of symbiosis. Fittingly, they turned their noses up at the sofa, each choosing instead one of the armchairs. Nick sprawled on his seat with his legs wide apart, arms spread across the back, very much the convinced macho man that, I later discovered, he actually was. Hannah didn't lean back but perched on the edge of her chair. She was, as it were, sitting at attention but at the same time appeared to be powerless. Time and again she glanced down at the baby. Otherwise, she was pretty much silent.

Nick was a muscleman with a continuous grin on his face that could easily morph into a winner's smile. His strong hands—go-getter hands—didn't give the impression of being used for gentle, sensitive stroking, although sometimes impressions can be wrong! Hannah had medium-length reddish hair that hung loose, and an incredibly delicate, long nose that looked like she should be balancing a pencil on its tip. A brief thought crept up on me about whether the little one fast asleep in the carrier also had saucer eyes. She certainly had her mother's hair color, as shown by what peeped out from under her summer bonnet. Maybe she would wake up during the session. My neuronal toggle for motherhood was definitely switched on, something I often find intriguing because I'm through raising children myself. Was Hannah still breastfeeding? She had such a slight figure, but an impressive bust.

My thoughts were abruptly interrupted as Nick quickly kicked off the discussion:

"Hannah doesn't feel like having sex anymore—and it's a problem."

His close-cropped hair stood at attention as if expressing the same resolution. It soon became apparent, however, that Hannah didn't want the kind of sex she could have with Nick. When it comes to reluctance, such subtle differences are important.

I asked him, "What do you consider to be 'good' sex?"

Nick's answer came out like a shot: "Well, the works—spontaneous, creative, in leather gear. In the old days, Hannah never turned her nose up at the idea. She was always ready to screw, anywhere." Sex became difficult after their third child was born, and now the fourth was here. The issue had been with them now for two years, which for people like Nick felt like a long time but for others is a mere detail. However, for me, Nick's assessment was important. He was unable to explain why his partner no longer wanted sex. For him it was inexplicable. He looked at his wife with an annoyed expression, the tone of his voice emphasizing his irritation. Obviously, he was not at all happy that Hannah wasn't as available as she used to be and that there was nothing he could do about it. I could understand him. Hannah was, in my opinion, someone who once had enjoyed stepping on the gas, reacting quickly to sexual stimulation, but who, sticking with the image, also had a normal—and for her, healthy—braking system. Physically overwhelmed by the many births and by her daily routine with the children, all exaggerated by having an insensitive husband, she had reduced her sexual appetite to what she considered to be a reasonable level. In doing so she had assumed power over sex in their relationship even if that was totally unintended. So it was not for nothing that Nick had the feeling that his wife was suddenly dictating their sex life. *She* decided whether a hug or a kiss became something more. He felt marginalized, stuck bowing to Hannah's wishes.

Did Hannah realize that compared to the early days she had taken her foot off the gas? Her explanation was "Give him an inch and he'll take a mile." To sidestep conflicts, she didn't allow her husband to touch her—a solution preferred by many couples for avoiding tensions but one that works only superficially.

"If only she would at least allow a French kiss," complained Nick the macho man (by now I was sure he was one).

I told him that a French kiss is also a form of penetration and that Hannah evidently, at that time, wasn't prepared to let him in.

In the course of our conversations it became apparent that the couple had very different ideas of what sex meant. Hannah couldn't have sex with Nick without first having some feeling of love, and Nick, on the other hand, couldn't show love before having had sex. That's how Nick explained it. I concluded that each of them needed both love and sex but in the opposite order. In the first years Hannah had adjusted to her husband, but at some stage her own needs had come increasingly to the fore. And she just didn't feel like getting into the leather gear that so turned him on.

"If you don't want to do it anymore like we used to with leather and all that stuff, then I'm no longer interested in you," he blustered.

Hannah looked at me as if she had heard it all before. With her look she was trying to provoke me into response. I did her a favor and asked Nick, "Did I hear you correctly? Your wife, on whom the whole house and family rely, should spontaneously get into leather gear just so you can get your kicks?"

Nick didn't even try to conceal his indignation: "I can't be bothered with vanilla sex."

"So just this kind of sex and nothing else?" I asked.

"Exactly!"

"Then welcome to the next ten years of abstinence!" I said to demonstrate the absurdity of his statement—and to provoke him. I got an ever stronger sense that he had never questioned his own needs. I added, "How is that supposed to work in practice? Hannah, after a long day's work with the kids, is then supposed to change into leathers for you? Just when the kids have gone to bed and she's exhausted?"

"Doesn't have to be evenings," said Nick. "I'm a carpenter. I can come home in the afternoons."

"Aha!" I replied. "And when Hannah saunters through the house in her leather outfit, you'll tell the kids that Mum's just playing Batwoman?"

"Yeah, something like that," he answered. He was able to love his wife only if she gave him enough sex. The Batwoman quip he ignored, but I think he wasn't particularly worried about the children finding out. He was only interested in his sex—a completely egocentric man. Remember the macho man from the bridge model? There's no space in his world for women and their needs, or for children.

Such men are not often guests in my love practice. Macho men don't stray into therapy as they seldom admit to having a problem. Nick had only agreed to therapy because he hoped it would "fix" his wife and things could return to how they used to be.

He was also someone who wasn't particularly well anchored to his masculinity. He was too tense and barely able to have balanced relationships with women. In order to pump himself up, he had to deprecate Hannah. Instead of choosing meaningful conversation, he went for coarse slogans. Nick should have considered himself lucky that his wife had gone along with his sexual preferences for so long without finding the space for her own requirements. But after the third child, she had felt that she was part of his life only when it involved sex—as if she was so small, almost invisible, and very easy to ignore.

For Nick, however, his penis must always assert his virile nature, be ready for action, so that he could assure himself what a great guy he was. No surprise, then, that Hannah's rejection endangered his self-image of manliness, provoking his sudden erection problems. These were certainly also bolstered by his age, his doubts about his masculinity, and the fact that he wasn't used to being turned down by his wife. Even when Hannah was prepared to have sex, Nick hardly ever reached a climax, or if he did, it was a huge effort. In an individual session later Nick admitted, "Hannah has to rub me long and hard." No wonder his poor wife was despairing! She may very well have been a red-hot vixen in earlier days, but since then her life had set her other priorities.

She sighed and said to her husband, "I don't want sex anymore without love. It's already been like that for way too long. To use your words, I just can't be bothered anymore." She looked him straight in eye. Her crimson hair suddenly seemed ablaze. She was pretty, and I could well imagine Nick wanting adventurous sex with her. At that moment she really did look like a scorcher.

"Do they actually love each other?" I jotted down in my notebook. I still had to find that out. The two of them had more stress than love in their marriage. I decided, though, to tell them in this first session something about stress and gender. Testosterone plays an important role in men's lives. This sex hormone, generally speaking, suppresses stress hormones (such as adrenaline and cortisol) and is released during physical activity and sex. Nick used sex to bring himself down. For him, it was totally reasonable to have sex before treating Hannah lovingly and in a relaxed way. For Hannah, however, oxytocin, the social bonding hormone, was the important one. Especially for women, oxytocin has a dampening effect on stress. Additionally, when women like Hannah spend the whole day with children and expend a lot of energy in physical contact, it's hardly surprising that gratifying their partners in the evening is not the first thing on their minds. Of course men too spend quality time with their children and oxytocin is released, but it doesn't have the same effect on their stress levels.

Hannah then asked, "Do hormonal differences in men and women determine the sex they have?"

It was a good question that is not easy to answer without a scientific lecture. That's why the short answer was "Not exclusively, but they're particularly influential when couples are suffering from stress."

My comments seemed to reassure them. Both Nick and Hannah were well aware that life with four children is not without complications. There was little time left for passion. At least they now knew that they could manage gender-typically and could tune in to their hormones.

At the end of the session, both were more understanding of their opposite number's problems—even the macho man! Finally they mentioned that in the following week they were going away on vacation as a family. I seized upon this information as a good opportunity to practice some exercises: awareness exercises, for which a bit of time is required. While doing them there should be no sex for roughly four weeks. Instead, time is scheduled for a mutual physical awareness program:

1. Breathe together in the spoon position for a few minutes.

2. Stroke the partner's back (fifteen minutes).

3. Stroke the partner's front (fifteen minutes). After Steps 2 and 3 are complete, it is important to exchange views about the experience and perceptions—first one person, then the other.

4. Finally, back to the spoon position, breathe together for a few minutes and then talk again about feelings and the experience.

For the person being stroked, this is all about being aware of the body without pressure, without having to do anything. All they have to do is enjoy what's happening at that very moment. The person stroking consciously and calmly explores their partner's body but at the same time notices their own feelings. Note: In the early stages, no touching the genitals!

After a while the rules are changed. In the next round, the genitals are casually included in the stroking exercises. Later, when couples are ready, the genitals alone are stroked. The rule change designates the stroking as foreplay, eventually leading to sex.

This exercise, developed by Masters and Johnson, should enable couples to make new sensual/sexual discoveries. I tend to modify the exercise depending on the needs of the couple in question. For instance, I let the person who is less passionate about sex decide when to move up a phase. I'm not dogmatic about it.

As for Nick and Hannah, I still maintain that you can't always expect gourmet sex; sometimes you have to switch to just plain cooking or even fast-food sex. I told Nick, "You should say goodbye to the idea of always having your special program or that everything has to be as you want it." And to Hannah, "Maybe, every now and then, you might feel like getting into your leathers." They seemed very fond of the idea of different kinds of meals. Nick grinned, but it wasn't a nixing grin or the old victory grin, simply a friendly grin. Well, that was definitely progress!

Two weeks later I received a text from Spain: "Skipped the third step and it was just good plain cooking."

I heard nothing from them for a long time, and hoped that they took time to talk to each other about problems. They had received new impulses from me and would come again if they communicated with each other honestly. The most important thing was to keep at it: initial improvements are no guarantee of long-term effectiveness.

Again ... or Still?

THREE YEARS LATER Hannah made an appointment to see me, this time without her husband. She sat in her armchair upright and attentive, again not leaning back, but something had changed, and it wasn't to be overlooked. Something good.

To begin with, however, she said that she was anemic and hadn't slept much, as Nick snored so loudly. Her days with the children were hard work, but she loved being a mother.

"And what is sex like?" I asked.

"We still do it, but not all that often, and mostly without intercourse."

"With or without leather outfits?"

"Without, because I don't like it anymore. Nick always says, 'You miserable bitch!' or 'I want to fuck you!' Sex is hard for him—his face gets totally tense. I don't think he feels much passion."

"And how do *you* feel?"

"I want him to stroke me, tell me he thinks I'm beautiful, that he loves me. I want something emotional, but Nick is incapable of that."

"I presume that you've thought about separating..."

"Unless things change, I don't want to grow old with Nick. He's like a block of ice that can't be melted. His toughness is deep—it's rooted in his soul. I'm beginning to think that he doesn't really want to feel *anything*. We can do as many awareness exercises as we want, but I don't get any closer to him. His life is geared to not wanting to feel anything. But I want to be with someone I can rely on emotionally." Hannah's cheeks had reddened slightly. I had never known her to string so many sentences together.

After a short pause she continued, saying that she still had loving feelings toward him, that she was happy for him that after years of struggling self-employed, he was now an employee and had less stress feeding his family. In this respect he'd become more relaxed, but not in his sex life.

"Could Nick come for an individual session with me?" I asked.

"I'll try to convince him."

After Hannah had left, I thought about how she had played along for so many years before she discovered her own path. Three years earlier, when they had first come to me as a couple, had they already considered the possibility of divorce? No—at least that's not the impression I had. They had become aware of this option more recently, maybe as the final consequence. Hannah had switched off. Nick, her husband, now really had to address his problems. If he didn't change his ways, his wife would leave him.

Nick appeared at the practice two days later. He had hardly changed in the three years since I'd last seen him, maybe just become a little plumper. Without being asked, he flopped down in the armchair where he'd sat the time before and launched in.

"I haven't got the faintest idea why Hannah's always jabbering on about love. We always used to have creative sex, sometimes in a hotel, sometimes in the ladies' room at a restaurant, in the forest, on tables, with kinky underwear—actually, we've tried almost everything." Before I could say anything, he continued his monologue: "I could have had any woman, but lately I can't even convince my own wife to sleep with me—"

"Have you actually agreed on monogamy?" I said, interrupting him. He obviously took the question to be a challenge to explain himself (false mind mapping).

"I'm not unfaithful," he replied. "Multiple relationships are too stressful. I wouldn't be able to concentrate on work."

"You've misunderstood me," I said. "I wasn't interested in whether you're faithful. But maybe it would be important to agree on alternatives. Let's leave that open for the time being."

Nick was once again already lost in his thoughts. "For five long years I've been bending over backward for her, and what's the result? Vanilla sex with my own wife! Sexually she's just left me in the lurch." He came across as full of hate. "She goes along with it just so I can relieve pressure. And I try my hardest to have an orgasm as fast as possible so she doesn't get tennis elbow. For four months now we've only been doing it manually. Not even one blow job.

Anyway, she never wanted that. Not anal, either. Fuck it! I have to really concentrate just to come."

Nick provided all the facts, and slowly I was able to get an idea of their sex life. The strained expression on his face that Hannah had described suddenly seemed to make sense. Nick didn't *enjoy* sex, he *performed* sex. I wanted to know more about how he masturbated. Maybe then I could draw other conclusions.

"I want to understand why everything's become so difficult for you. Can you tell me exactly how you masturbate? How do you handle your penis?"

"Why?" Nick muttered. "Just the way it's done!"

"Can you be a bit more precise?"

"Okay, then, in the middle."

"And with how much pressure?"

"Pressure?" he asked.

"On an imaginary scale of one to ten—one being very soft, ten very hard—where would you place yourself?" This scale is subjective, but it can give therapists an indication of the pressure used. I demonstrate high pressure by almost tucking one finger into the base of my thumb. This almost always means that the client feels less than it's possible to feel. Low pressure I demonstrate by fluttering with one hand over the back of the other like a butterfly or by gently rubbing a finger up and down. Afterward I let the client demonstrate with his own fingers the amount of pressure he uses. Sometimes I give him a pen or some other long object as a penis model.

Nick thought for a little while and finally said, "Somewhere between six and seven."

"Is that really enough for you to come?" I had reckoned on a higher number and suspected that he wasn't being honest with me as far as his arousal was concerned. I told him that.

"You're right," he said. "Before I really come, I have to put a dildo or a finger up my bum to stimulate my prostate gland."

"Do you rub your penis?"

"No, I just squeeze it, in the middle!" He then grabbed a pen from the plastic coffee table and showed me the relevant place.

"When you're masturbating, do you have a particular picture in your mind?"

"I come on breasts."

"Any other fantasies?"

"No, always strapping, massive tits!"

The sex act itself was not part of his sexual fantasies. (Chris the fitness freak was the same, remember?) Likewise, he wasn't particularly loving toward his penis. Up till then, he hadn't thought of it as a feeling and communicating organ.

It would take a vast amount of convincing before he would seriously believe that other and new ways of handling his penis and the rest of body would be of enormous benefit to him, mainly for relaxation but also for emotional purposes. Many men simply can't imagine the benefits. Nick and many other male clients find the thought of doing exercises boring.

"And what about porn?" I asked. Nick said that he regularly watched hard-core movies on the internet and that they aroused him. There he could find what he was missing with Hannah—these women did what they were told, they played along.

"And anything else you want from sex?"

Nick didn't need long to think about it. His dark eyes lit up. "It would be really cool to make my own porn movie."

"And what would it include?" I wanted to learn more about his secret desires.

"A whole lot. Oral sex, her and me. Intercourse, anal and vaginal, also dressed. Licking everywhere, but no whips—not really my thing. Kissing, of course, and plenty of eye contact."

Nick's ideas were actually not what you could classify as unusual sexual fantasies. For many people, that would be a reasonable program. His sexual system was beginning to make sense to me, and I asked myself what he meant by eye contact—it sounded almost like love.

As if he could read my thoughts, he explained: "Actually, I'm someone who needs harmony. More so than Hannah—she's confrontational."

I quietly asked myself whether Hannah perhaps tries to place unpleasant things on the table in order to clear them up while her husband prefers making a wide detour to avoid conflict. I expressed my thoughts. Nick was continuing with his own thread, though, as he suddenly blurted out, "Generally, I can't love a woman I have sex with."

That was a confession. I translated it as: The client cannot link his genital sensations (below) with his emotional ones (above). But was I right? Three years earlier he had claimed that after sex with his wife, he had loving feelings toward her and was able to show them. His statement didn't seem to match reality. This also became even more apparent with his next remark: "Though when we have sex, something merges for a while."

"You're contradicting yourself!" I told him.

I got the clear picture that the ideas in Nick's head didn't tally with reality but that he didn't notice this. A blind spot? What didn't he want to see or couldn't see? Did love hurt him? Did it trigger fear? What did he really feel or think? There would be no way around these questions.

On leaving he said, with unfocused eyes, "Hannah and I just have a marriage of convenience."

I was sure there was much more that needed to come to light. Did it make any sense for them to remain together as a couple? Or was separation the best option? I prescribed another session, with both of them attending.

Two weeks later, Hannah came alone. She told me that Nick had moved into one of the children's rooms, that he simply wasn't able to tackle his problems. I could understand that she didn't like the situation and also felt how sad her husband must be.

Nick came to the practice four months later. He had moved out of their apartment and was living with a single friend. He saw Hannah from time to time but had hardly any contact with the children. At least he and Hannah weren't quarreling so much. She didn't want separation or couples therapy.

"And what do *you* want?" I asked.

"To learn. To show more emotions. I want to be the man that I could be. I do try to push it all aside, but I'm beginning to understand the interrelationships."

I made my point clear. "You do realize that you're a proper macho man, don't you?" While saying this I smiled. He took my comment calmly and said, "I just don't feel any emotions."

That was probably the heart of the matter. Every healthy person can feel emotions, but you can learn to ignore them. That's the bitter truth.

It was an honest confession by Nick. With this kind of openness, I could begin couples therapy.

But the next appointment was never made.

I don't know how the couple are doing today.

13

Be My Echo:

NARCISSISM IN
RELATIONSHIPS

MODERN THERAPISTS DON'T see clients as wounded souls or victims. They know about people's resilience—that people can endure unbelievable hardships and still rebound. This is why I leave the responsibility for clients with the clients, and do so with a great amount of respect. I don't consider myself to be someone who guides and leads. I don't tell anyone which path to take but figuratively remain two paces behind them. This, as I mentioned at the beginning of the book, means we're still on an equal footing.

For many decades, clients (and patients) lay on the famous dreaded couch—so, literally, lower down. In this position it is clear that a very different relationship develops between client and therapist. In my office, I can look clients directly in the eye and vice versa. Body language and eye contact are highly relevant to therapy, especially in discussions about sexuality. Also, reading each other's thoughts eye to eye (mind mapping) can happen normally.

Clients, however, in the process, calculate the therapist's next step, usually at the speed of light, and arm themselves inwardly against anything they feel could become unpleasant for them. The good thing about this is that when I'm able to read them, I can tell where their difficulties lie. Most clients quickly lower their defenses, open up, and participate. But for some the anxiety is so great subconsciously that they are unwilling to accept anything that comes to light at all. They shut themselves down: no confessions, no scrutinizing of problems. To put it simply, they are people with mental disorders related to early childhood bonding. They do come to the practice with sexual issues, but they bring with them additional problems. Sex becomes the sideshow—it is solely a symptom or reflection of an impaired capacity for forming relationships.

Therapists have a wide range of instinctive or conscious practical tricks to get such patients through therapy. It's sobering for me as a sex therapist to realize at a certain point that a problem cannot be solved by couples or sex therapy. Many of these clients are already undergoing psychiatric treatment and, in principle, it is right that when being advised about sexual issues they seek competent help elsewhere—for instance, from a sex therapist. But sometimes that simply doesn't work: the real central disorder keeps pushing into the foreground, and work on sexuality becomes tricky. Then I no longer consider that mine is the right address for such cases.

This became particularly clear to me with a certain narcissistic client addicted to sex who, every day, sought the services of prostitutes and who, as a high-income broker, could offer generous rewards.

"I get horny when I see a woman's bike," he said when he came to my practice for the first time. Björn was in his mid-thirties, with white-blond hair flattened by gel and a preference for blue shirts. Although he was in therapy with a psychiatrist because of his pronounced narcissism and had made steps in the right direction—he had come to understand that he was a narcissist and had learned a few new and useful behavioral guides—his sex therapy had foundered because his sexually inexperienced wife, Miriam, was way out of her depth with her husband. Miriam was a tough businesswoman. She had recognized her husband's narcissism early on, knew all about his compulsive visits to prostitutes, and was having trouble accepting this, although she had tried very hard. But sexually, she was a late developer and still insecure. Her relationship with Björn didn't really improve things. Every time she felt brave enough and bought sexy lingerie (white!) and began to get excited about wearing it, he managed to ruin everything with one poisoned remark: "And *that's* supposed to turn me on?" He had no idea what he was triggering.

His thoughts: *Black is hot!* Only *black.* My thoughts: *Inability to empathize—that's a typical narcissist for you!* Miriam didn't have much sexual desire for him (and how could it be any other way?). Sex with Björn was clumsy, and she thought, probably correctly, that she had to act like a prostitute to satisfy him.

Clients like Björn always seem to me to be lacking something, and that's the way it is. Certain behavior patterns, like "building a trusting relationship," "appreciating someone else," or, in a positive sense, "getting the feel of someone"—basically, just "being human"—weren't sufficiently instilled in them or learned by them during childhood. Fundamental connections are missing in their brains, to put it flippantly: the framework for being a sensitive human isn't available. This was the case with Björn, whose problems were so deep rooted that sex therapy wasn't able to help him much. When Miriam had to go to a special clinic for treatment for a serious psychosomatic illness, which I was not surprised to hear had worsened, we decided to end the therapy.

In Greek mythology, Narcissus was a handsome youth who was able to love only himself. Having seen his reflection in a pool, he immediately fell in love with it and, on trying to hug it, fell into the pool and drowned. The woman who loved him was called Echo. Metaphorically speaking, Narcissus' story means there is only one relationship mode that works for a narcissistic person: the partner has to be a reflection of himself, his echo. This is what the next case is all about. The couple are Anne and Joel.

Ascendant ... Eel

JUST TO MAKE things clear from the start, Anne and Joel also broke off therapy. Despite a fair amount of success in the early stages, it became increasingly apparent that narcissistic Joel was able to read me quicker than I could read him. I spent much time discussing with myself how I had failed to establish clear rules from the start. Joel managed, almost playfully, to maneuver me into the same defensive, hamstrung position in which he had trapped his wife, Anne, for years. In a fraction of a second he had everything under his control. His pronounced egotism went hand in hand with his incapacity for self-criticism. At the same time I was sure that although it sometimes looked as if Joel was playing a power game, in reality it was just a survival strategy.

The problem with Anne and Joel, or so it seemed from what they said at the beginning, was that they hardly ever had sex. Anne said she felt tired and just didn't feel like it. When he wasn't allowed to have sex at home, Joel got bored and wanted to screw elsewhere, preferably every day. This demand was initially on the back burner during therapy. Both agreed that the point of the therapy was to increase Anne's sexual appetite. So the couple had given me a clear mandate.

Anne, a tall, slim woman with curly hair, was in her early forties. Joel, with a shaved head and a gangly elegance, was a bit older. They had got to know each other after "a large number of other partners," as they put it, so both were sexually very experienced. Since then they had become the proud parents of three children. Anne didn't use contraceptives, and Joel used tadalafil, an impotence drug, so that he could use condoms. (Time and again, the same little details appear on the table!)

When Anne said during a session, "I feel like it in the afternoons," Joel asked with a grin, "And at what time?" So it seemed to me that both their gas pedals were fine. But why was Anne braking? I soon received the first hint.

"I'm not fixated on having an orgasm during sex," Joel exclaimed, probing me with his gaze.

And I fell for it: I saw a chance of backing him and agreed with him on this point—at last, a man not interested only in the Great Orgasm Hunt! So, yes, I told him that it's certainly not always only about having an orgasm. I had the feeling, however, that with Joel something else was resonating, something I didn't want to accept. He tried to manipulate me to get me on his side—a classic example of narcissistic behavior. But instead of raising the issue, I moved on to another subject.

He noticed this mistake of mine, and knew that I had circumvented something. He noted this inwardly at once, adding it to the list of my weaknesses that I was pretty sure he kept mentally. Part of my strategy, as with all clients, was to cautiously build a stable relationship with him and then later to jump into the troubled waters. Unfortunately, with narcissists this usually backfires. If I don't immediately show that I can read him, he will think—correctly—that he can't trust me. I should have shown Joel my true motives right from the start: that I would very much like to understand him but that he can't play around with me like he does with his wife. Instead, I had provided him with a reality in which he could do just that.

The therapist's expression for this is the *co-construction of reality*. The client explains or says something, and the therapist lets it stand even though it doesn't reflect the professional realities or, for a variety of reasons, fails to match the content. Or the therapist leaves things unnamed or lets them slip through, as I did with Joel. And then all of a sudden this therapeutic contribution manifests a reality that actually should have been corrected and treated. The therapist co-constructed.

A simple hypothetical example: A man who has not had sex with his wife for sixteen years, because she didn't want it, thinks about having an affair and comes to me beforehand to ease his guilty conscience. The man says, "What else can I do? If she doesn't want sex with me, I have no other choice." As understandable as the thought is, I still can't find it good. A therapist can't let something like that go. If we do, we are reinforcing an objectively false reality. I would prefer to see him admit to his wife that he is no longer willing to spend the rest of his life without sex and that a solution has to be found.

Back to Joel. In his case, I could have said to him, "You're looking at me as if you want to know whether I agree with you, but I'll leave that aside for the moment. I'm much more interested in the reason why you are *not* fixated on orgasms."

Joel had tested me, and if it had been a game of points, the score would have been 1–0 for him.

But then Anne jumped in, and my feeling that this was about something deeper was confirmed.

"True. Sometimes he stops in the middle of it even though I would like to come." She even upped the ante: "By the way, he launches a kiss offensive when he wants sex, and often gets too close in the process. Luckily, he's often away on business. I can recuperate when he's not there."

Joel watched his wife and let what was said stand. Obviously, he had nothing to add.

This behavior was borne out in the course of therapy. Joel was a true artist when it came to evading issues. He was unable to blame himself and to take responsibility for his influence on the relationship. His main objectives were to keep control and to deflect feelings of guilt. He was also unable to admit weaknesses. He was always slipping away from me. And he had perfected the art of sidestepping issues.

My assistant, Anita, who has a way with words, would say of him: "Ascendant ... eel!" and actually that's not too bad a description. Time and again I tried to convince Joel with watertight arguments, but as soon as the situation got a bit tight, he managed to wriggle free with a single sentence.

Joel, speaking of their daily routines, told me that his wife was simply unable to keep any of their joint decisions. "Anne has no commitment."

I doubted that the decisions were joint, and was right. He and Anne had simply not agreed.

"I don't want to just function," she said cautiously.

"I'm not in the mood for your reproachful undertones," countered Joel, and suddenly looked at Anne almost hatefully. "Then I'll just go somewhere else for sex."

They quarreled furiously about their household arrangements. Anne described how Joel always wanted everything planned out minutely; even the children suffered from his need to control.

Joel retorted, "She just doesn't get it! She simply can't keep things tidy. The fridge, for example—it's supposed to be filled perfectly, everything on the agreed-on shelf, and the agreed-on amounts of everything so we can plan meals for the next days. But Anne just can't cope. That's why I give her shopping lists!"

In between, Joel tried to give me orders: if he wasn't going to be allowed to interrupt his wife (which he continuously did), then at least I had to let him finish speaking. The same rules for everyone. I explained to him that in my practice, an important precondition is that we *don't* have the same rules for everybody. Just the opposite: my rules are the only ones that apply, and they depend on the situation—if only because clients want to change something that's failing when they use their familiar way of coping with problems. For the rest of the session, Joel was upset and sulked. There was tension in the air, and it was obvious that he didn't agree with my viewpoint. This he let me know at the slightest opportunity—I had to restate my opinions and again became defensive.

Nevertheless, work progressed, as did the couple's project to enhance their sex life. They learned something new in the sessions that followed. They were having fun, and discovered a new refuge for sex—their old camper, parked in a remote corner of their property, a farmhouse outside the city. In the camper they were away from the children, and all of a sudden sex between them was in full swing and, lo and behold, for Joel, right now, I was the greatest.

"Oh, Ms. Henning, it has *never* worked out as quickly as it did with you." Before me, there had already been six "bad" therapists and Joel paid my fees for eight more sessions without even being asked.

When considering his compliments later, I noticed a few things. First, in the narcissistic image that Joel had of himself, he deserved only the best. This included his therapist, so there I was. Second, with his gushing praise he was testing whether I was prone to compliments, whether I was vain. While praising me, he once again had an alert, probing expression on his face. And again I had fallen for it, had co-constructed. Had I replied with "Oh, thanks" and carried on with the session like a professional, I would have shown him that I couldn't be flattered. Sadly, I was proud of his compliment, and I'm pretty sure I showed it—easy prey for Joel, who was continuously scanning me for my strengths and weaknesses, sounding out my procedures and strategies so that he could be better armed against me and against the danger of being hurt.

His compliment served to get me under his control. His high opinion of me would exist only as long as I complied.

Termination of therapy was, in principle, already programmed. It didn't take long before I was no longer the greatest.

But at this stage, Joel and Anne were still coming to the sessions.

The Therapist as Client

YOU CAN ONLY be a good therapist as long as you are able to differentiate yourself. The therapist's stage of differentiation, their personality, probably has the greatest effect on treatment. This means the therapist needs to know their own motives and weaknesses.

I used to tend far more toward unconditionally wanting to help a client than I do nowadays. I would become defensive or sometimes even get into arguments with clients who rejected advice that I was offering. True to my nature, I wanted my honesty and intentions to be understood and to a certain extent appreciated, too. Joel saw through that. He sensed that I wanted to be right and that I wanted his recognition. This gave him power over me, which played right into his need to control.

When I tried to form an opinion of him and to substantiate it by questions or suppositions, he smelled the danger—the loss of control—immediately. Mistrust sharpened his awareness like a predator scenting its prey. He then suddenly switched to eel mode. My feelings: *Whoops! I'm walking on eggshells!* I became more cautious ... unfortunately. This too Joel, always on the lookout for more control, noted and exploited.

All this quickly came to light during the third session with Anne and Joel. I opened up the office door and when

Anne took off her light spring jacket, I noticed something small, black, and square dangling from her neck.

"What have you got there?" I asked, bewildered.

"I sometimes record things," she answered while hesitantly watching my reaction. She went on to explain that she needed a recorder at home as she sometimes had to prove something to Joel by playing his own words back to him. Judging by her expression, she did indeed feel a bit embarrassed, but apparently they had both agreed to tape our session.

Joel stood next to his wife and seemed to find the whole situation completely normal. He said, "When Anne can prove me wrong, I'm sometimes willing to admit it."

Once again I had my doubts. You hardly have any chance against a narcissistic personality even with a tape recorder. If something is going wrong in the relationship, someone else is always responsible, with or without evidence. My suspicion was that by taping their session, Joel wanted to increase the control he so urgently needed. Time and again in the previous sessions there had been questions about who said (or didn't say) what, and I had allowed myself to get involved in the discussion. All the same I had begun to pry open his narcissistic system and had shown him several times that—irritating as he was—I still upheld a relationship to him. Instinctively he felt that my office could become dangerous for him.

I didn't allow the session to be recorded. I explained in a friendly tone that I didn't want to fight and that without any doubt he would win. I would prefer having a conversation where we bring out the best in each other.

But with narcissistic clients, you have to be confrontational, almost to the limits of tolerance. Otherwise, there's no effect. They need the truth, coupled with regard. I have to be plain and clear without being debasing, moralistic, or aggressive. With the last of these I have problems. Years ago David Schnarch told me during a pause in a seminar, "When therapists are differentiated and mature, they can impart the same content with a different degree of delicacy." And I'm working on just that. Practicing therapy every day, you do indeed touch on a number of essential issues. Since then, I have to admit, my work experiences have made me gentler.

I was also able to empathize with Joel. I tried to show him how relationships and emotions work, commented on situations and correlations so that he formed new images of reliability, of being loved and accepted, so he could move a little bit away from his cravings for power and control and open himself up. This, of course, necessitated him not breaking contact with me.

Every behavioral pattern and every emotion has its sound reason. With Joel it was chiefly about his childhood disappointments, about his anger and indignation. It was important for him in relationships that these feelings were appreciated—no matter what happened. It was just a shame that Joel couldn't admit to the sadness that lay beneath these feelings. It would have triggered too many fears of being rejected.

In this third session I was a little more successful in keeping Joel in line. There was even a sense of slight progress. At the door he thanked me for "putting up" with him—a true compliment. But was it said with affectionate familiarity? Or was I again just the "best therapist in the world"?

A Sneaking Feeling

THE PERSON I was most worried about, however, was Anne. At every visit she looked at me as if I was her last chance. She mostly sat there quietly, observed, and listened. Sometimes it seemed as if I was reading a plea for sympathy in her eyes, as if she were saying, "Look, it's that difficult with this man. I don't have a chance." Yes, I could feel it in my bones.

Whenever I turned to her, I would notice how clearly she saw herself. She also mentioned her own faults. When I asked her how long she could continue living with all these rules and obsessive tidiness, she thought for a long time— Joel, for a change, didn't interrupt. Anne gave herself still more time to find an answer.

"And?" asked Joel eventually, irritated that it was taking so long.

Anne stared at the floor. Again she remained silent.

I tried putting it differently. "What reasons are there to have sex with a man who treats you like Joel does?"

Anne rocked back and forth on the sofa. With each movement her recorder knocked against her chest. She was wearing it again for this, the fourth session. (It had become her constant companion, although it had to be turned off in my office.) I read the answer in her eyes. Anne had huge difficulty standing up for herself, and not only with Joel. I made one more tiny little attempt at explaining to her what was happening inside her, and I think it helped.

The result was that Joel felt he was being harried by *two* women, and he couldn't be persuaded that this wasn't the case. He was outraged, called me a "bad therapist." Nevertheless, it was a good session as Anne had been able to see herself in the web that her husband had spun. Her only chance of standing up to him, in my opinion, was to bolster herself using her own powers. But this could (or would) just end in separation.

The point of therapy, however, couldn't be for Anne to learn from me how to be an even better echo of her husband. She was right in withholding sex if she didn't desire Joel anymore. Internally she was in a raging fury about the whole situation. Her main emotion, however, was sadness, a great sadness.

In a solo session with me, Anne noticed that I made no secret of knowing how miserable she was. "I know we have to separate," she said out of the blue, and began crying.

"I understand if you can't—or at least can't just yet," was my reply.

In relationships like Anne and Joel's, both parties are scared of losing each other. Joel handled his fears by treating Anne abrasively and disrespectfully, and in doing so kept her at a distance, not really letting her get close to him. He was guaranteeing that the amount of pain should she leave him (and subconsciously he was reckoning on this happening at any time) would then not be too severe. Hurt and abandonment were his earliest experiences.

Anne's fears of splitting up, on the other hand, led her to turn a blind eye to certain things that she didn't want to see and to a certain degree, even to deny their existence.

In the fourth session things escalated. I forced Joel into a corner with honesty, recognition, and affection, and he was barely able to cope with the emotional closeness for even a minute. But I wasn't going to let go, and continued to aim closer. His inner tension was high, and Anne's wasn't much less.

When Joel left briefly for the restroom, Anne was worried and questioned me about the intensity of the argument.

I told her, "It wasn't an argument. I just don't always agree with Joel's point of view. We go over all the tiny details so that he can learn to accept gray areas without fear. Otherwise, there's only black and white for him."

On returning, Joel told me that nobody had ever treated him like that and that he liked it. The next day, however, he canceled all the remaining appointments by email. He asked me to pay back the fees for them, which I immediately did. While Anne and Joel had been on the way out of what proved to be their final session, I had told Anne loudly and clearly that she was very welcome to come alone to a session at any time that suited her. I wanted to let them both know that in that session we had reached an important point at which Anne had been honest about her situation—even if it was only for a moment—and had obviously felt good about it.

In the end I wasn't able to help Anne and Joel. We had simply begun to scratch the surface.

Neither of them came again. Since then I haven't wasted a lot of time mulling over terminating therapy. There are clients who don't want to be or can't be helped. And when I hear the compliment "Ms. Henning, you're a wonderful therapist—we wanted and got the best!" it's highly likely that next time I won't look quite as happy and may very well say, "Maybe I won't be able to help you. After all, you're actually a pretty tricky case."

14

Desire Chooses Its Own Path:

FETISHES, S&M, AND MORE

IMAGINE THAT YOUR husband gets sexually aroused by feathers. By plastic sandals. By a chair with a naked woman sitting on it. Or a particularly knotty one: by flatulence. More than likely he has a fetish. Sexual desire has many ways of manifesting itself. You may be polygamous or monogamous, prefer bondage or vanilla sex, go through life as an exhibitionist or as a voyeur, love people of your own sex or of more than one sex. Desire is not bound by limits.

But first of all, back to fetishes!

According to the older definition, a *fetish* is an object believed to have magical powers. But it can also be an object that invokes sexual arousal in people. The International Statistical Classification of Diseases and Related Health Problems (ICD), published by the World Health Organization (WHO), adds that a fetish is an "inanimate object." The foot, well known to be arousing to quite a large number of people, doesn't belong to the fetish group according to the ICD definition—at least not when the foot belongs to an animate person. Strictly speaking, it would be considered a fetish only when linked to necrophilia, a sexual preference focusing on dead bodies! Most of the foot fetishists I have become acquainted with, however, would be put right off by that thought. In my experience, an animate foot can certainly be classified as a fetish just like many other body parts. Some medical descriptions are actually a bit far-fetched—or simply old-fashioned.

The Magic of a Fetish

I AM OFTEN asked how fetishes start. I consider fetishes from a conditioning perspective, the result of acquired experiences of sexual desire. In childhood or adolescence, an object or behavioral pattern can become associated with a sexual experience, often through some sort of defining key event. It could be a shiny red raincoat worn by your mother's friend who, when visiting, looked at you lovingly, or a black cape wrapped around you when you had your hair cut for the first time and the sweet hairdresser (seen in the mirror) ran her fingers through your hair. Both can trigger an erection, or at least a feeling of sexual well-being.

It could, however, also be the hot blast of water hitting your body while taking a shower together with a girlfriend after she spent the night at your parents' house without any adult knowing. Some men can explain precisely how they arrived at their fetish.

And yes, it is mostly men who have fetishes. Much thinking has gone into why this is, but there have been no real solid scientific answers. One explanation, however, could be that men, on getting an erection, find it easier to connect their arousal to a certain event or object and that this association makes it easier for them to develop a fetish.

For centuries fetishism was considered an illness or disorder. Someone with a fetish was seen as sick or perverted. To some degree this is still true nowadays. Doctors saw (and see) in fetishes a failure in sexual preference, which counts for them as a personality or behavioral malfunction. If we are to believe the WHO, exhibitionism, voyeurism, frotteurism (sexual arousal by rubbing against a nonconsenting person), sadomasochism, and sex with animals are sexual disorders.

Societies provide the context in which it is decided what is abnormal, perverted, or even criminal. There are hardly any scientific or medical reasons for declaring certain sexual behaviors to be pathological. The people found "guilty" are those who are "different" from the "majority." Gay people who like holding hands, for example, would be well advised not to do so in Moscow's Red Square, even nowadays. It wasn't all that long ago that gay people were criminally prosecuted in Germany, where I live—homosexuality was only decriminalized in 1973. The ICD stopped classifying homosexuality as an illness only after 1992. As a Russian edition of my book *Make Love* was being planned, the publishers asked whether the pages mentioning homosexuality could be omitted. This I categorically declined.

Sexual norms can vary significantly in different cultures and countries. Women in some Muslim countries, such as Afghanistan, who have affairs or premarital sex have to accept the risk of being stoned or even killed. Such deeply anchored moral and sexual perceptions have an appalling potency even today. They were and still are being used to keep people, especially women, under control.

More customs, more nonsense? In Denmark, pedophilia is forbidden, but not the founding of a club for like-minded people to meet. Many times this has led to outrage in the media but not to any changes in the law. Incidentally, sexual acts with animals are not forbidden in my home country.

My own opinion about all this is clear: everything is normal and should be permitted, as long as no one crosses anyone else's boundaries or harms their dignity, as long as it is consensual (the WHO speaks of "conscious agreement"), and, of course, as long as the participants are having fun! For me, only sex with children or animals is taboo, and unfortunately these are more common than people realize. In these cases, the sex partner is not in a position to consciously agree, and it is precisely this conscious agreement that, for me, is the bare minimum of all acceptable sexual interactions.

Your average Joe or Jane, however, often sees things differently. People are frightened of things they don't understand and often reject them out of hand without much thought. It is hardly surprising that problems often accompany the sexual variances of those concerned, which is also a reason many practitioners remain guarded about their fetishes. Particularly with fetishists, their own partners frequently know nothing about their secret passions, and the shock is all the greater when after twenty years of marriage a hidden box of gas masks, chains, or black leather gear is discovered together with the latest copies of magazines like *Heavy Rubber* or *Marquis*.

More than a few of the men with fetishes who have come to my practice have been exposed this way by their partners. After their discovery, these men's partners have trouble understanding and even more trouble tolerating their husbands having to arouse themselves "abnormally." As a result, sex, which in most cases had still been taking place (in addition to the fetish), is denied. The men, correctly, feel judged, begin to question their actions, doubt their mental health, and come up with a dire diagnosis: "I'm a pervert." People know exactly when they deviate from a norm and the effect this could have on their lives should it ever become known. For most people the fetish is not the problem—rather, the problem is the marginalization.

Couples in which the partner has found her husband "guilty" often come to an arrangement (mostly unspoken) whereby they no longer discuss the subject. They push the fetish out of their lives and instead install taboo zones in their relationships, causing enormous pressure.

But what meaningful actions can you take when your partner is sexually aroused by a fetish? Should you split from him? Do you give him the chance to fulfill his needs elsewhere? For someone with a tendency to s&m, for example, "somewhere else" could mean going to a dominatrix. An appointment with a dominatrix could be viewed as the most harmless form of being unfaithful, as it doesn't usually involve intercourse or love. A visit to a "mistress" who knows her job is probably as safe as going to the hairdresser or massage therapist. In the end everyone makes their own decision about what is and what isn't dangerous. But you have to be aware that not many people are able to voluntarily break their fetish because that would mean an end to the sexual arousal that the fetish brings. Nobody likes surrendering something that appeals and that easily stimulates.

When they are not able to use their fetish, many fetishists suffer from functional sexual disorders and have difficulty desiring their partners. Others, however, curse their fetish and would give anything to be rid of it because it controls their lives and becomes almost compulsive—particularly if it's forbidden.

Catwoman and the Dental Technician

MAX WAS SIXTY and had been married to Sabine for thirty-seven years. They knew each other for three years before taking the plunge. Max was just over six feet tall and slim, and his once dark hair had thinned out and become gray. He was a dental technician and his lab was next door to his wife's nail studio. Max described himself as very quiet and deliberate. He loved working alone on the artificial teeth until everything fit. He often forgot to take his lunch break, becoming aware of it only when one of his assistants set something to eat in front of him. He and Sabine had two grown children. The last time they had sex was ten years earlier. Max had come to my office because his wife had discovered something in the attic that she wasn't supposed to discover, namely, his playthings: clamps, whips, and hand-cuffs. Early on, right at the start of their relationship, Max had tried to interest Sabine in his "toys," had even bought her a book on the subject, but in vain. She wasn't interested in the slightest. Eventually, peace returned. From then on they simply had "normal" sex and pretended nothing had happened. They often had disagreements about sex—Sabine wanted more—but all in all there were no further noticeable occurrences. The situation began to escalate only when Sabine found Max's cache.

"It was a dumb mistake that my wife discovered all my things in the box," said Max.

"What are they?" I asked.

He immediately knew what I was referring to. "I'm a sub, a masochist, who likes to be dominated. Back then, when I explained it to Sabine, she thought it was sick and perverted. I had already been to a dominatrix."

"And apart from this you get on well together?"

"Well... my wife has a memory like an elephant. She can remember things I've long since forgotten about. She uses this to get me on the defensive." He sighed. "Actually, you'd think that that might appeal to me, but she makes it all sound so accusing. And she's not particularly frugal with her accusations."

"What's her main complaint?"

"She thinks I'm a self-indulgent egotist. Maybe because I don't pay the attention to her needs that she'd like me to. I can understand her, that she's annoyed about it. She wants more sex, more hugs."

I asked Max whether he could persuade her to come for a solo session so I could form a better picture of the situation. She was the one who had sent Max to me. Still, it could interest her to speak to me herself. And it did. She made an appointment for the very next week.

When she arrived at the office, one phrase immediately sprang to mind about her appearance: well-groomed. Fingernails artificially extended and painted poppy red; hair with plenty of body; stylish high heels and a skirt and blazer of the finest quality. For my tastes, she had been a bit over-generous with the perfume, but really just a bit.

"When I first met my husband, we were roughly twenty," she explained. "He said at that time that I could beat him if I felt like it. I didn't feel like it. And later we never spoke of it again." She was obviously calculating how many years had passed, and I gave her time before she pressed on. "At some stage he moved out of our shared bedroom. That must have been about fifteen years ago..." She said this as if she herself was amazed that everything had been so long ago, that it had got that far. She consoled herself with the thought that Max snored and she needed her sleep, so everything was okay.

"About five years ago I found Viagra in the guest room that had become my husband's bedroom. 'What does he need Viagra for?' I asked myself. I assumed that he indulged his cravings elsewhere. I consider my husband to be very egotistical."

There they were again, the accusations that Max had spoken to me about.

"Do you want a divorce?"

"Not at all. I just want us to be honest with each other, not to fight anymore. I want nothing more than him to become loving again and tell me what's wrong with him. I just don't understand it—we're just a regular couple, aren't we?"

Two weeks later I had the next appointment with Sabine's husband—or he with me. As soon as he sat down on the sofa, he was grinning.

"I found my wife's sex toy," he said.

I let his remark stand without comment. Instead I asked, "Has something changed between you?"

"No. As always, she lectures me. I should say something, start talking to her. I've been thinking it over for ages, but whether I lie or tell the truth, it's bound to hurt."

Well, at least he was confronting the situation.

"Do you like only S&M or other sex too?"

"I like normal sex just as much. My fetish is just another variety." Was he being truthful? I did indeed think that Max favored his "other variety."

"What will happen to your marriage if you keep your fetish?"

"I don't want to give up S&M, and I don't want to give up my wife. That's my dilemma."

I couldn't have put it better.

They both came to the next appointment.

"My head is just full of chaos," Sabine said in a flurry. This time her fingernails were dark red, almost black. Matching her mood? "I sense my feelings for my husband shrinking from day to day. This S&M business just makes me sick. Max tried to explain it to me, but I still don't get it."

Max felt misunderstood. He couldn't comprehend why Sabine had these feelings of disgust.

"What am I doing wrong? At least I'm not cheating on you," he pleaded. "And anyway, I can't buck the fetish. I'm completely at its mercy," he added. "Even if I wanted to, I couldn't suppress it."

Max's remark about at least not cheating on her certainly felt different for him than it did for her. Did she maybe fear that one day it could come to that? Cheating on her with someone who would do it right?

"Perhaps you could explain it to me again in a bit more detail?" Sabine asked in a tone that implied a certain amount of criticism, but even more dominant was her desperation. "I imagine all sorts of disgusting things."

At last the moment had come when Max could talk about his arousal, in the sheltered confines of my love practice. Except he didn't. Something was standing in the way. Slowly I was beginning to understand Sabine's exasperation. I too wanted to get Max talking and to tell him that it was far less dangerous to talk about his fetish than not to. But I had already noticed that Max, when put under pressure, sat there like a young child who had to invent an excuse for his mother. It was all a bit awkward, but with his crooked grin he hoped that Sabine would think him cute and innocent and maybe even a bit cheeky. In this case, he had definitely deserved punishment. It was as if this time there wasn't a handbag as substitute husband next to my client but a third "person" who had suddenly arrived, one who also had to be questioned from time to time, namely, Max's fetish. He just couldn't quite get it out of his head, which confirmed my suspicion that it was probably more important to him than he was admitting.

Sabine didn't take notice of all this. She had begun to compose herself a little; she wasn't interested in destroying anyone; she just wanted to understand. "Just let me finally find out what I'm saying no to—who knows, maybe then I'll say yes." She didn't let go. She wanted to discover whether her disgust was justified or not. Maybe everything wasn't as bad as she had imagined. "And why do you need Viagra, Max?"

"To masturbate," he confessed.

The answer put Sabine at ease. Max was apparently worried about not having an erection when he needed one, which was a more plausible reason for avoiding intercourse. Had he become clever through experience? In any case, he obviously had erection troubles when masturbating, though masturbation almost always worked out better than sex with his wife. With her it was not only the pressure of his own expectations but the pressure of hers, too.

Even though these conversations progressed haltingly at first, they weren't in vain. Max and Sabine reported that they had been on long walks together and had had a lot to say to each other. They had begun touching each other again, and it was a beautiful feeling to feel naked skin again. They patted each other on the behind and kissed—things they hadn't done for years. But they hadn't yet slept together.

Two months passed before they returned to the office. I heard pretty intriguing things. Max and Sabine had been on vacation and one evening, they emptied a bottle of wine, talked a lot, and spontaneously decided to play a bit. At the beginning she was his slave and he led her, with a collar and leash, across the floor of their little wooden cabin on a remote azure lake. Both were completely naked. Their game amused them so much that they could only laugh. Sexually, they weren't aroused in the slightest. Afterward, Sabine forced Max to chop wood naked while she looked on from the porch sipping a cocktail. They had found the ax in a little woodshed attached to the cabin and it had given Sabine the idea. And it continued: Sabine tied Max to the lawnmower, which they also found in the shed, and left him there in the dark while she enjoyed a foam bath.

The "official" reason for this measure was the logs that Max had chopped were too big and he had to be "punished for this at all costs."

"If I need you after my bath, I'll come and get you," she told him. "In the meantime, make sure you keep that erection up for me!" She gave him a stern look and felt that it was giving her quite a bit of satisfaction.

"You could also beat me afterward," he said with a trembling voice.

That was going too far for her, but it gave her another idea.

"No, as a punishment I will *not* beat you! You haven't earned that yet."

Sabine's plan worked, and afterward they had perfectly normal sex. (Whatever that may be—anyway, on that evening for Max and Sabine, there was no fetish involved.)

After their experience on vacation, Sabine suggested buying wigs, patent leather boots, and a black catsuit. They found what they were looking for in a sex store, and even a couple of bondage films ended up at the checkout. After that the couple had sex more frequently, even though Sabine still wasn't all that keen on her husband being submissive or on tying him up.

"I always think that he's missing the pain, and I can't give him that." Still, she was able to concede, "There's something to it, though. At least I can vent my anger at Max."

Max looked at her as she was saying this with his crooked grin. That got me to thinking about how I would get rid of my own husband if he got on my nerves. Tie him up tight and shove him in the broom closet! Release him only when necessary—for sex!

Although Sabine didn't share her husband's tendencies, Sabine and Max had demonstrated something important:

there *is* a way of living with a fetish as a couple, at least to a certain extent. For Sabine it was important that her partner be honest with her, and thus she was able to overcome her initial feelings of disgust. For his part, Max was increasingly able to open up and to reveal precisely what it was that aroused him.

"Well, nowadays I can imagine going with you to an event like that ... ," said Sabine. She meant a fetish party.

"Shall we watch a couple of dirty movies tonight?" Max was in his element.

What many people don't realize is that fetishes almost always happen in the head: they're all about emotional arousal and fantasies. These men automatically become tense, both emotionally and physically, when they are dominated. They become scared and, in doing so, hold their breath. Neither is particularly conducive to circulation in the penis or to lusty thoughts involving sexual intercourse with a partner. The sexual fantasies in a fetish revolve not around actual penetration but solely around the fetish and the emotions associated with it. Many people with a fetish say that the penis is not especially important in their thoughts or to their physical sensations.

As a sex therapist I work at making these emotionally laden men better acquainted with their genitals, move attention down below to anchor onto and normalize their thrusting virility. (Generally this involves the same exercises I used for early ejaculator Alan.) If we succeed in increasing awareness and feeling in the genitals, the client usually arrives at the idea of wanting something to do with his penis. Gradually, the fetish fades into the background, where it can still act as a particularly arousing fantasy. Max only had to *think* about his fetish for his arousal to be catapulted to lofty heights.

Thus the general objective isn't to make the fetish, which has worked well up until then, disappear completely, but rather, and more importantly, to increase the sexual spectrum so that sexual desire isn't exclusively focused on the fetish.

Under the Makeup Table

ANTON, A CLASSICAL guitarist, was in his mid-thirties. He hadn't had sex with his wife, Eva, for a year and a half. They had no children but did have a huge, unapproachable Siberian cat. Eva, a dark beauty with a long ponytail, was almost ten years older than the skinny, ash-blond Anton, but you wouldn't notice it right off.

Anton's parents had been actors at the local theater but had retired. However, it seemed to me that Anton's mother wanted to continue her career through her son. She stuck to him like superglue, though she had been living with her husband hundreds of miles away for many years—a significant factor, as we are soon to discover.

As a child Anton had spent countless nights at the theater under his mother's makeup table while she prepared herself for her show. He sat between her muscular, nylon-stockinged legs, and there he found the two smells that he began to love: her sweaty feet and his own full diapers. Anton would stay there, always in semi-darkness, until, just before the show started, his nanny gathered him and put him to bed. Every time he was miserable, he missed his mother and screamed and lashed out wildly. After he started school, he was sometimes still allowed to creep under the makeup table but was annoyed about having to go home before the show. He no longer screamed or lashed out, but he still hated being separated from his mother.

Now Anton was sitting on the couch with Eva, who was fine with his sweaty-feet fetish and was even prepared to play along with it. But the "thing with the shit" she would not or could not tolerate. Anton had developed not only foot and smell fetishes but also an excrement fetish—and, on top of this, very particular thoughts about them. About his foot and scent fetishes he said, "The feet should really stink! But only the feet. Never the intimate areas or the armpits." He didn't shower often: he, of course, saw body scent as a good thing. Ankles he also found highly erotic. But the best thing was still big feet, preferably in high-heeled shoes. His mother, he explained, wore a European size 41—a U.S. size 10.

What made things more difficult for Eva was that Anton's mother was literally sitting in front of him every day while they Skyped for hours. During the Skype sessions, Anton performed guitar exercises that his mother had set for him while she listened. Eva said, "His mother is always present, calls constantly. Anton can't do anything to counter it." The couple had been discussing the situation with Anton's mother for years. One time Eva came out of the bathroom with just a small towel around her hips and heard the penetrating voice of her mother-in-law from the music room: "You should put something on, sweetheart—it's not spring yet, you know." Obviously, Anton's mother had spotted her on the laptop camera. Since then Eva had shut the doors and crept around the apartment even when Anton wasn't Skyping. She felt she was being watched.

"Do you enjoy playing guitar for your mother?" I asked slightly ironically.

"I've already told her I don't want to be a classical guitarist," Anton replied. "Mama definitely wants me to carry on." When he said *Mama,* the stress was on the second syllable. It didn't sound like he felt small and dependent, but he continued to practice guitar with Mama. Did he realize that his marriage was at stake? He had developed a sensory disorder in his fingers and could no longer feel the guitar strings properly.

As for what Anton's sexual system looked like . . . Remember the four spheres? Evidence suggested that Anton was only minimally interested in his penis; it was practically irrelevant. He didn't like fellatio, so no blow jobs. If he ejaculated at all, he came too quickly. "My penis isn't an organ of pleasure," he told me one time. He utterly dismissed the idea of holding his penis differently, in a better way. For him, rubbing his penis wasn't sex, and if it went on for too long, the penis just went limp. I can't say it often enough: the penis is not a machine. The older you get, the more it needs loving attention.

In addition, Anton's fantasies reflected his sexual system—a woman who wet herself or who practiced "controlled crapping." He had asked Eva many times to use the toilet for and with him. She told me that she did it with him two or three times and then it just got too much for her.

Everyone knows the strange pleasure of having to wait and hold back before emptying the bowels. When we're children, this involved jumping around and squeezing. In the process, the muscles of the pelvic floor contract, and there's a pull in the stomach and the genitals. But doing something just for your partner when you have absolutely no feelings of arousal is, of course, difficult, just like it was for the dentist and his catwoman. To Anton, this restraint was linked to his sense of security beneath the makeup table. There he was, in his "cave" with his "fragrant" sodden diapers and a grandstand view of his mother's legs—a secure, cozy world.

Anton now understood his sexual system but admitted that he couldn't afford the therapy. "Still, after today's talk I feel less perverted and my wife is also relieved," he said on departing. I had my doubts as to whether this was really true. Eva didn't look too happy when they left the office. My thoughts were that their problems were far from solved.

The Exhibitionist Who Wasn't

JONATHAN LIKED BEING naked. Even as a child he had enjoyed undressing in front of others. He came to the practice because he was worried that his inclination was getting increasingly pronounced. He was very concerned about this, and his wife definitely was not to discover it. As a result he lived a double life. At home in the bedroom he was a normal lover (that worked out, albeit without being particularly exciting); outside of his own four walls he felt he was an exhibitionist, although he told me quite plainly that he didn't want to be one.

After the first half hour with Jonathan, however, I wasn't at all sure whether he was an exhibitionist in the normal sense of the term—that is, whether he became sexually aroused by exposing himself to others or by being watched while performing sexual activities, which can also be characteristic of exhibitionists. I wanted to clarify this uncertainty and discover his sexual system's setup, the interaction of his four spheres. Not all clients are right in their self-diagnosis.

After Jonathan discovered his tendencies as a child, he went through a number of phases, but he was always ashamed when he noticed how good he felt when he was naked in front of others or when he even thought about it. It was hardly surprising to hear that he had already been to four or five other therapists before coming to me. It was a heavy burden for him that his sexual preference was so little tolerated by others, and in that he was right. After all, according to the WHO classification, exhibitionism, if we stick with his own diagnosis for a while, is a personality and behavioral disorder.

Jonathan was what you would describe as gangly, with arms and legs that dangled awkwardly from his body. His light ginger hair was slightly too long and already thinning, and he had a face full of freckles. In younger years he could have been mistaken for a male Pippi Longstocking. He gave his age as forty-four on the registration form.

"As a child, you liked undressing in front of others, but were you aroused when you did that?" I asked.

"I can't really remember exactly, but I don't think so. It was more like a kind of a game, out of curiosity . . . like playing doctor."

"When did you begin to find it sexually interesting, then?"

"In my mind I have a very particular memory. I had driven to the beach with a friend and we were lying on our towels. We must have been about fifteen. When my friend ran into the water naked, all of a sudden I got an erection. It had nothing to do with *him*, that's for sure. I'm not interested in men in that way. The whole thing was seen by a woman who was nearby and staring down below rather primly. I was totally ashamed and lost my erection almost immediately."

"What was so bad about it for you? And what had aroused you in the first place?"

"Where I grew up, it was perfectly normal to be naked at the beach, but in that situation it was about something completely different—I didn't want the woman to think I was interested in men."

"What caused the erection, and what was so good about it?"

"That she saw me?" Jonathan answered my question with a question, as if he wasn't entirely sure.

"Maybe it was just the relaxation, the warm sun on your skin, a general feeling of well-being?" I suggested. "That would have been absolutely normal for an adolescent in puberty."

This information seemed to get Jonathan thinking, and I left him in peace for a while.

"And what happened next?" I asked eventually. Somehow I couldn't imagine Jonathan exposing himself to people in the park or just wearing a trench coat in a shopping mall, and even less so now than before this part of our conversation.

"Somehow I get fun out of being looked at," he began before telling me about changing after gym class. "Our small group of friends would compare our penises. That was great!" But there weren't only positive experiences. One summer he played with a friend naked in the garden and they sprayed each other with a garden hose. "That was fun, but the next day in school my friend, who had a big penis, told everyone how small mine was. And he told them I had been circumcised. The very same day everyone ogled at me in the showers after swimming class. That was terrible." Nevertheless, after a while Jonathan discovered that he kept getting an erection when he noticed people looking at his penis.

"It all happened pretty quickly back then. Nowadays it takes much longer to react," he said sadly.

"Who did you expose yourself to?" I persisted. "Did you go to parks?"

"Good God, no! I sometimes tried at a swingers club, but it was the wrong place . . . They just put up with me. I'm so ashamed about it—I just don't know what to do. I've even tried prostitutes that I paid to admire me."

He spoke not for the first time about his need to be admired, but most exhibitionists want to shock other people. Other people's anger then triggers their own arousal. Is it possible that Jonathan was more interested in having his penis judged than in having it exposed? Did he simply want to know whether other people admired it? Shocking victims was definitely not on his agenda.

"Have you already tried exposing yourself to your wife?"

"I once tried masturbating in the tub, but she reacted as if she was bored and looked away."

Somehow that wasn't exactly an ingenious attempt to win over his own wife.

"Does your wife have even the faintest idea about your tendency? Have you ever talked to her about it?"

Jonathan nodded. "I asked her once, 'Do you like my penis?'" There we were again with the need for admiration and appreciation. "But she didn't want to talk about it, and after that she didn't even want sex."

He admitted that what he wanted out of that situation was that Lena look him in the eyes and say, "Yes, your penis is beautiful! Absolutely incredible!" Jonathan, however, had not realized that she couldn't possibly know what was going on in his mind. Or could she? Was she just pretending not to know what was happening?

The more I let him talk, the clearer it became: Jonathan's thrills were emotional; they were happening above. He enjoyed touching himself, admittedly, but penetration or ejaculation were not particularly important to him (some of you must recognize this). So there was a definite division between "upstairs" and "downstairs." When I confronted him with my theory, he said, "Purely emotional, not genital? Yes, you could describe it as that." He preferred to fantasize about standing around in a changeroom with other people and how excited and aroused he got from taking his clothes off.

Jonathan was always wondering where he could appear naked—the park was, as before, not an option. But the more he tried not to think about his fetish, the wilder his thoughts became. And so did the fears that his fantasies could get out of hand. This was understandable. In 1989 the now late Daniel Wegner, a professor of social psychology at Harvard, researched the extent to which suppressed thoughts affect our psyche. Wegner was inspired by a story from the life of Leo Tolstoy. Tolstoy's older brother gave him the task of remaining sitting in the corner until he wasn't thinking about a white bear anymore. When after a few hours the brother returned, he was amazed to find the young Leo still sitting in the corner unable to banish the image of a furry white animal from his mind. Wegner recreated the thought experiment with his students. The assignment was again "Don't think about white bears for the next five minutes." All the students failed. The experiment proved that forbidding thoughts has the opposite effect. It is a paradox.

For an experiment we performed when I was a student, I had to walk through a room of my fellow students and we had to imagine that we lived in a country where it was forbidden to look at feet. It was less than thirty seconds before I desperately wanted to look at feet. The more I tried not to, the more intense the feeling became in my head and upper chest. And my feet got cold. In the end I had to stand in a corner of the room and stare hard at the wall in front of me so as to not be tempted to look at the other students' feet. This seemed to be the only way to bear the situation, and I was hugely relieved when our teacher ended the exercise. At long last I was able to give all the feet around me a good look!

For Jonathan there was only one way to solve his dilemma. He had to find a way of integrating his wife, a way of persuading her to verbally admire his penis. I was pretty sure that he could live with his fetish—in my eyes he wasn't an exhibitionist—if he could talk about it with her. Some partners say without being prompted, "I love seeing you naked. I adore looking at your body." Or, "Your penis is awesome, I love it, and omigod isn't it huge!" But not Jonathan's wife—maybe because she read him right long ago and knew how sensitive the subject was for him, and thus also for her.

With our sessions, however, Jonathan began to feel less out of place with his disposition, which made him think much more often about having the dreaded talk with Lena—it might really offer a proper chance for him. One day he plucked up the courage, and lo and behold, it worked. He found out in the conversation that his wife had known about the situation for a long time but that she hadn't dared mention it because she felt embarrassed. As they continued to speak, the atmosphere gradually eased. They agreed that Lena, every now and then, would go into the bathroom when Jonathan was taking a shower to "admire him" or to ask him to show her his penis. Maybe one day soon she would even enjoy looking at his "stiffy"! Watching it getting bigger and bigger the longer she looked at it. People who take risks often win more than they ever could have lost.

15

Sex and Gender

RECENTLY I WENT to the hairdresser's, to Toby, who a couple of weeks earlier had become the father of a cute daughter. He was bursting with pride. We were talking about this and that when all of a sudden he asked, "Why can't women accept praise? When we pay a client a compliment, she'll almost always dismiss it with something like, 'You have to say that to make me happy!' "

I thought I understood what Toby was getting at and said, "Exactly. A man would just say thanks."

Toby managed to top this and guided me to the genuine man's world by adding, "No, a man would just say: 'I know!' "

The difference is real.

A couple of years ago I met the American couples and family therapist John Gray. Gray has written comprehensive studies on the differences between the sexes. What makes a man? What makes a woman? Is there a formula? Gray wrote a book in the early '90s that went on to become a bestseller: *Men Are from Mars, Women Are from Venus.* Mars and Venus are planets, but in mythology they also represent different forces—the god of war, Mars, and the goddess of love, Venus. Gray described the male powers as potent, strong, and purposeful, while in contrast the female powers he characterized as softer and more evenly balanced. These two powers, according to the therapist, are complementary, particularly in partnerships and in sexuality. Gray's book was a kind of user's manual for helping men and women find a way through the stormy waters of modern relationships and for understanding the two genders' communication forms. Regardless of stereotypes, I enjoyed reading the book, and it was written entertainingly. When it comes to clichés, each society creates its own.

Up until then I hadn't met Gray personally, but that was to change in Copenhagen, where we were both attending a conference. During dinner with other colleagues, mostly sexologists, the topic of discussion turned to views on the increasing numbers of couples considering their partners as friends rather than sexual partners. The other therapists' comments I can't exactly recall, but Gray's remarks stuck with me. He explained how he used to believe that men should become softer and show more emotion and that women should become more assertive. Then Gray said, grinning, "There were strict traditions. There were stipulations about how a 'good' man or a 'good' woman had to be. We therapists wanted to retaliate, we wanted to soften the gender roles. To achieve this we demanded, among other things, that men learn to knit and crochet and that women pick up hammers from time to time. To this day I still have a guilty conscience because the women eventually came to me alone and said, 'So, now we have two pussies at home!'"

During the '80s and '90s, many therapists had the idea of reeducating the genders. Basically not too bad an idea: it was, so to speak, birthed by feminists and nurtured by the women's movement. As a result, in the hard struggle of the sexes, to some extent, two groups of losers were produced— one, Mars women and Venus men; the other, couples who hardly ever had any sex. The sexual tension between the sexes got left behind. Of course there were and still are plenty of reasons to fight for women's equality, particularly in the sexual domain (without question, but not the topic here).

I too had always found it difficult to accept that in trying to achieve equality, both sexes had to renounce or abandon their specific behavior patterns or needs. Men and women live with both Mars and Venus tendencies. Each person knows best how feminine or masculine they feel, irrespective of sex, and they find partners with whom they can have exciting sexual relations. I tried to bring up my son, who was born in 1993, to show and care about his emotions. As we all know, big boys don't cry, but I taught and showed him that as a man, you can cry or do whatever else you want to do to show how you're feeling at any given moment. He and many of his friends can now admit to mistakes and show emotions, including by crying, without feeling that they have surrendered their masculinity and will be considered weak. Maybe these men are even thought to be strong and genuine precisely *because* they can be "weak."

John Gray once said, "Women from the baby-boomer generation don't respect their husbands." And there is some truth in it. Men of today live in conflict. Should they be "new men" or macho men? Baby-boomer women, generally, are allowed to be strong and can compete with men. Men, on the other hand, have to keep a lower profile, learn to understand women, and to question their sex. In a number of ways, many lose some of their status and masculinity in the process. It is not necessary to take up crochet for this to happen (think about Alan, Shayne, and a number of the other men in this book).

In 2015 I was invited onto a talk show together with two crocheting policemen who had been invited because of their "unusual hobby." It seemed to me that we were taking part in a trial of gender equality. Had they been policewomen, it wouldn't have interested anyone.

Still, things have happened. Women with welding equipment are no longer ogled at in disbelief (unlike crocheting male cops). And in the September 2016 edition of the Swiss journal *Das Magazin*, I read an article by Denise Bucher, Anna Miller, and Kerstin Hasse on how "emancipation had blurred the lines of the idea of what constitutes femininity and masculinity. Maybe misunderstandings are just the price to be paid on the path to a more open, equal society in which there are no clear role allocations, no strict specifications about what it means to be a woman or a man." It's true: today, partners in relationships define themselves as individuals. Everyone tries to profit from their partner, to improve their own self-esteem, and to feel more complete. We have yet to find out whether this is the better path.

A number of my clients, however, are more concerned with the feeling of being born in the wrong body or of having a sense of gender that doesn't match their outward appearance. Some belong to the 10 percent of the population who prefer sex with a partner of their own sex. This is still conspicuous. Where it all can lead we are about to find out.

Still Missing the Words

SOME PEOPLE FEEL that they live in the wrong body. Conventional medicine uses the neat term *gender dysphoria*. But have you ever considered who decided that there should be only two genders? Or decided which gender belongs in bed with which? Maximilian Probst wrote in 2016 for *Zeit Online*, "The choice of gender categories is staggering," and went on to list some, including androgynous, bi-gender, gender variable, genderqueer, intersexual, and transgender, "Where earlier you had two genders to choose from, there are now sixteen!" he said. "And that is a wonderful thing, but it's also a huge challenge." It looks like the world really is changing.

In Norway, legislation was recently passed allowing children to decide their gender for themselves without medical or psychological assessors, with the consent of a parent. It is a "historic step," as the Norwegian health minister Bent Høie said. In 2017, Germany officially acknowledged third-gender options. Laws like this can also benefit people who genetically, anatomically, or hormonally cannot be conclusively classified as female or male. Some of these intersexual people discover their particular biological sex very late, maybe even notice that they feel "different" by chance as adults. An example: a man had hot flashes and went to see his doctor. During the examination they discovered that he had ovaries and a partial vagina. The diagnosis was that he was in menopause! Nowadays, things are considered more carefully than in previous decades when, if in doubt, everything "unnecessary" was simply chopped off.

One day a woman who had been born in a male body and had undergone many gender reassignment operations came to my practice. She was married to a man who was living in a woman's body but who hadn't been through any surgery. Outwardly they looked like a lesbian couple and would eventually, if he went through with the surgery to make him outwardly the man he was, appear as heterosexuals. Categorizing people into clearly defined genders is sometimes less than appropriate.

My client Annette was in her mid-thirties and wore a Chanel-like blue and white suit. Before surgery she had been very near suicide. Suicide rates in the transgender population are very high: according to a U.S. survey, 41 percent of transgender people claimed to have already tried to kill themselves. The suicide rate for the population as a whole is 1.6 percent.

"How can I picture it? What does it feel like to be born in a different body?" I asked Annette.

Annette smiled and stroked her long, straight hair. "I stand in my kitchen making a sandwich and ask myself, where do these big hairy male hands that are fumbling around and actually have nothing to do with me come from?" Her voice was bright and friendly.

She earned a living working for the rights of people like her. She supported early use of corrective hormone treatment, before puberty kicks in and forms the body permanently. In her case, this was not a possibility. She had to consciously attempt to make her voice sound higher, and she will never lose her angular facial features or her Adam's apple.

When I was talking about Annette's case with a friend, anonymously, he asked me, "How does your client actually know what it feels like to be a woman?"

I answered, "How do you know you're a man? Because visually you match what you feel? Feelings are real. You don't have to explain them." Still, I tried. "Does your penis feel part of you, or do you think of it as alien? Do you like your beard? Aha, you're nodding. If you were in the wrong body, you would probably want to chop your crown jewels off with a kitchen knife, dress in skirts, and put on makeup. It's not just a fixed idea! Just like it isn't a fixed idea that you know for sure that your penis belongs to you." He then understood.

The 2015 biopic *The Danish Girl* is about the first known case of sex reassignment surgery (male to female) in the world, in the early 1930s. It's a poignant movie: the patient dies after the second operation, but at least as a woman. The phrase *sex reversal* is often used for the operation, but the correct term is *sex reassignment,* as the physical appearance of gender is reassigned to the felt gender.

Almost everyone has difficulty at first when their partner in a longtime relationship declares their sexual "otherness." I have often heard of men who for years have been true to the role of a heterosexual married monogamous family man even though they are gay. For women, it mostly isn't so much of a problem coming out as a lesbian, which is possibly down to the fact that gay men in our society have had to bear more hostility in the past than gay women have.

If my partner were to become attracted to men, there would be only one reaction on my side: "Let's stay friends." A relationship just wouldn't be possible if he no longer felt a sexual desire toward me, if he wasn't interested in the woman that I am. On the other hand, if he were bisexual, then maybe he would *also* be attracted to me.

"Am I Gay?"

FERDINAND, FORTY-EIGHT, WAS a sales rep, and consequently often away on business. The three words that sprang to mind when I saw him for the first time were *dynamic*, *athletic*, and *attractive*. His wife, Alexandra, with whom he had three children, was a year younger and definitely weighed twenty to thirty pounds too much. She looked unhealthy but seemed agile and curious. Once they had settled on the sofa, Ferdinand confessed: "I'm now *almost* sure that I'm gay." The uncertainty about which sex Ferdinand preferred seemed to have dulled his natural liveliness somewhat. Alexandra, on the other hand, was simply sad, as she had long suspected this to be true. Both said that they planned to remain together.

In the course of our discussion, Ferdinand repeatedly said that he wanted a solo session with me, and we arranged one for the following week. The remainder of the first session was spent going over the couple's past, the time before Ferdinand's problems became apparent.

When he came alone and sat down on the sofa, he said, "I've gotten to know someone I lust for. I get butterflies in my stomach, and if I repress it, I'll regret it later. Everything is so much better with him—kissing, hugging . . . I've never experienced anything as intense with my wife. I want to stand by my feelings, and I want to separate from Alexandra."

Wow! Within a week what used to be uncertainty had become a definite decision. That was quick! Or was Ferdinand not being entirely truthful? He later explained that he really wasn't certain for a long time. After the three of us talked, he had felt a kind of license. On returning from a short business trip, he had gone to a sauna and immediately met someone. Ferdinand's eyes lit up.

I asked him, "When are you going to tell your wife?"

"As soon as possible. I want to move out of our apartment. At long last, I want to be human again."

Bit by bit I began to learn more of the background. Ferdinand had first slept with a man four years earlier, and as a result he and Alexandra had gone to a therapist: for Ferdinand it was unthinkable that he could ever sleep with his wife again. The therapist showed them some exercises that were intended to get them physically reacquainted. And with some success: they were having sex again. Ferdinand enjoyed it too, but he couldn't shake off the feelings he had had for a man, couldn't totally wipe out the memories. They were still smoldering. He kept telling himself that he was a family man, that he couldn't allow such escapades. Nevertheless, naked men in the shower aroused him. It was almost as if he was still in his youth.

Ferdinand's father died young, so he and his seven sisters had to grow up quickly. He suspected that his mother had sensed his sexual orientation early: she told him off a number of times and attempted to turn his attentions to girls. Ferdinand took a long time to find his first girlfriend. He didn't have the opportunity to try things out and spent a long time only masturbating. He did it into a sink—a speedy, neutral act without thinking concretely about men or women. His first proper experience of sexual intercourse was at twenty-four, with an experienced woman. The relationship lasted about a year. He didn't feel like sex for many months after they split up, until a year later when he met his next girlfriend. He never thought that his sexual system was simply saying no to women. He excluded men as sexual

partners. At thirty he married Alexandra, and through his
three children and his marriage he defined himself as a
family man, just as his father had been. He did have sex,
but he never would have claimed to be really aroused by
Alexandra. He only experienced arousal after he met that
man in the sauna and suddenly began imagining a relationship with him. Since then they actually had started having
a relationship and saw each other almost every day.

So was Ferdinand gay?

For me the answer was clear: Yes, he was gay. He didn't
need to say anything more to me. His body had given him
the answer. Now he only had to talk to Alexandra about his
identity.

"I Just Can't Seem to Find My Place"

VONDA TOOK UP a lot of space when she strode into my
office. She was in her mid-fifties, had a tomboy haircut, jeans, lumberjack shirt and tank top, and walked
through the room like a cowboy, plumping herself down
in a chair with her legs wide apart. A graceful crossing
of legs? No chance! Without further ado, she got down
to talking about why she had come to see me, and in a
deep voice said, "I'm neither one nor the other. My whole
life I've been thinking about my male and female sides.
I never felt like other women, *proper* women. When I
was younger I was even harder and more manlike than
today. Since menopause started, things have gotten
better."

Wow! What an entrance! Vonda really had spent a lot of time considering her situation.

"Do you have sex with men or women?" I asked.

"I started out having sex with men, then when I was twenty-six I switched to women. I just react sexually much more strongly to them. But it took a great internal struggle to accept that. It was pretty complicated. Now I have sex only with women. But for a number of years it was almost every day, since that was what my then partner wanted, but it's never been really satisfying."

"What was unsatisfying about it?"

"Sex as such isn't so easy. I have a really big clitoris that sticks out and up, like a little penis. Even when I'm walking, it prickles," she remarked. "That's why I only wear baggy pants, like a man." For the last part of the sentence she grabbed her crotch and laughed. She had a good sense of humor that definitely had helped to make her life easier—and as she told me, she couldn't be aroused via her breasts.

For me as a sexologist, her remark about the size of her clitoris was very interesting: it could provide clues as to whether Vonda, as far as her hormones were concerned, was possibly made differently from "typical" women. Hormones aren't responsible for everything, but they are responsible for quite a lot. It seemed like Vonda was somewhat geared toward masculinity, and that this "somewhat" was the cause of her problems.

"Do you masturbate?" I asked bluntly.

"Rarely. Somehow I just can't do it. Only when my partner comes, then I rub and press until I eventually come too. It's pretty exhausting—the orgasm is short, almost like nothing, and after there's no feeling of pleasant relief."

Gradually I was getting the impression of why Vonda was dissatisfied with her sex life, and based on her account, I was sure that she was very tense when she tried to reach her climax. I asked her to describe "pressing" in a bit more detail.

She told me it was more like thrusting, just like men do, and went on to explain how aroused she would become when she watched men masturbate. She was fascinated by the penis and had often wondered what it would have been like to have a proper one. (Well, she did have a *kind of* penis.)

"Do you use sex toys?" Many lesbians use dildos for penetration, and I wanted to find out whether Vonda favored them.

"No, don't like them," she answered categorically. Her rejection was related to what's called *female receptivity*—the wish to absorb something, to be penetrated, which is part of the archaic essence of being a woman. I had the impression that we should be talking about Vonda's feelings about her own gender.

It's difficult developing a full and beautiful sexual sense of self when you have trouble aligning yourself with a particular sex, when you permanently feel somehow wrong. Vonda evidently tended toward masculine behavior, as witnessed by her total rejection of the dildo. She clearly stated that she didn't want to be penetrated and that she was aroused by thrusting and pressing; not only her behavior but her whole presence and being reflected masculinity. Penetration wasn't only something that she rejected for herself but she also wasn't interested in penetrating her partner—with fingers or dildos.

Six years earlier, at forty-nine, she had fallen deeply in love. She met Marianne, who was then almost seventy. The two women had independently booked a biking vacation in France.

"Marianne was a real athlete. In comparison, I'm a lazybones," Vonda told me. From her words I could deduce that

they became a couple. During long evenings by the camp-
fire they got talking, and eventually Vonda admitted to her
new acquaintance that she was beginning to feel something
for her. Marianne reacted cautiously, saying that she wasn't
a lesbian and also that she had a husband, children, and
grandchildren.

But a couple of weeks after Vonda's confession, Marianne, who lived some two hundred miles away, phoned
her. Despite the distance and the fact that Marianne
wasn't a lesbian, a tenderness had developed between the
two women. They met again and had sex. For Vonda, the
touching and cuddling were things that her feminine side
induced. Her early sex had been mostly mechanical. Her
relationship with Marianne became an epiphany of love.

"You're still together," I said—more of a confirmation
than a question.

"Yes, for six years. We see each other for three weeks, and
then not for three weeks. We keep our own apartments and
our own lives. Marianne's still afraid that a family member
will find out about our relationship. She's divorced now, but
her children aren't allowed to know."

"Is that a problem for you?" I still wasn't really sure why
she was here at all.

"Not in the slightest. I finally feel like I don't have to
struggle, I've arrived. And I have time to myself."

"But there's something . . . ?" Cautiously, I sounded
things out.

"Sex—I have no desire for it at all."

Sex therapists distinguish between lust and desire (as
opposed to libido, which is merely a reflex in the pelvic
area). Lust is an emotional perception; desire is where lust
leads. But what is desired? An orgasm? Being loved? In any
case, at least theoretically, there is desire for both love and

sex. In sexology, these can be described as twin columns, right next to each other, and on top of them—the roof, as it were—relationships are held in place. I let Vonda first describe what love means for her.

"Genital and emotional are very different animals," she said, agreeing with my example as if she could read my mind. She made a clear distinction between "upstairs," the desire for love, and "downstairs," sexual desire. As Vonda was about to itemize, things like respect, shared goals and values, rituals, trust, communication, appreciation, faithfulness, mutual consent, and even material security all belong to the "love" column. All in all, it could be put succinctly: "Me, in particular!" This column also includes some aspects of physicality, like tenderness, kissing, cuddling, or touching someone's skin.

"But you *are* desiring, then," I said, contradicting her. "You want closeness and love, you want to blend in with your partner, and you can do all that without sex. These are different and perfectly normal desires."

Vonda looked at me thoughtfully, then smiled.

The column of sexual desire, in contrast, stands for physicality that is distinctly sexual and genital. Reflex stimulation (libido) and eroticism are also found here. Many couples begin sex in the "love" column, with gentle caressing, and hope that the bridge to the "sex" column will appear all by itself. This often doesn't happen; more likely, someone will fall asleep. Sex therapists have to keep coaxing people back to the sexual. Otherwise, there's a tendency for clients to get stranded in the "love" column, very often as best friends. I always take a good look at how couples are placed in both columns. Sexual contact is very different from tender caresses. There is a want behind it, a desire for something, an intensity. The partner can feel the difference. When someone bows out of the "love" column, the relationship is over. When the "sex" column starts to crumble, the relationship, under some circumstances, can still be maintained (although this is often associated with one partner being unfaithful). For Vonda, anyway, there was no question of ending the relationship. She had merely bowed out genitally. Her column of sexual desire was in the process of collapsing, but her column of love was still rooted and intact.

"It's still possible for you and your genitals to make friends again," I said, quietly adding, "and in a way that you've probably never gotten to know them before: exclusively as the woman that you also are." My feeling was that Vonda could learn to stop thinking of her clitoris as a little penis and think of it as something that could be full of pleasure for her, as the center of her femininity. Maybe she could even discover her "within," her vagina, as an area that could be aroused.

Vonda nodded and told me that there wasn't much of a "keyboard" on her clitoris, just a very small spot that did the trick, and she could even pinpoint it, which she proceeded to do with a drawing.

I said, "That's precisely what I meant: you should extend your keyboard and start playing the whole instrument instead of just one or two keys." So we would be working in the Physiological Sphere and would gradually see how Vonda's feelings about being a "proper" woman changed (Perception Sphere).

One of my other considerations would have meant dealing with Vonda's method of arousal. (Again in the Physiological Sphere: How exactly can I boost my arousal?) Then, once her arousal levels had improved, a certain desire for new, good, intensive genital feelings during sex might emerge (this taking place in the Perception Sphere). And when Vonda discovered how she liked it, she could teach Marianne how to touch her.

We agreed on ten appointments. Vonda wanted to come every other week, and we got down to work a short while later.

Half a year later was the final appointment, and I could hardly believe my eyes. To mark the occasion, Vonda arrived in a short skirt. She had super legs, and I told her so.

"I know," she answered.

16

What's Left to Say

A T THE SAME time in the '50s as the Kinsey reports on human sexual behavior were causing a stir around the world, a book called *Hvordan, mor?* ("What's That, Mom?") was published in Denmark. The book consisted of eight fictional conversations between five-year-old Peter and his mother about questions of sex. It was written by Sten Hegeler, who, together with his wife, Inge, almost ten years later published *An ABZ of Love*. There was a huge outcry at that time as *An ABZ of Love*, both linguistically and visually, was very explicit in handling sexuality. Hegeler commented, "If someone says something that everyone thinks is wonderful, it's accepted, but you didn't really need to say it then, did you. If, on the other hand, someone says something that goes against the grain, then maybe things can begin to move." I always find that these words bring back disquieting memories. I too have been publicly attacked, several times. Among other things, because of my educational work I have been accused of making children sexually aware too soon, and told that this is dangerous—even sometimes when working with fourteen- to sixteen-year-olds!

The fact is that from the very beginning, children are sexual entities. Sex education doesn't mean only telling adolescents in puberty to use condoms; it's more about the small things that have happened long ago, some of which would happen all by themselves if they were only allowed to. Sadly, most parents find it difficult to admit that their children could possibly arouse themselves sexually, have fun with their own libidos, and find pleasure in their own bodies. They prefer to think about their offspring's innocence and purity. But children *are* interested in their bodies, including in sexual ways. At the beginning, children are their natural selves, and because of this they end up touching their genitals almost incidentally and very soon after that discover how much fun it is. Already at eight months babies begin touching themselves consciously and the feel-good factor grows for them.

Precisely for that reason we parents should learn to talk about sex so that we can answer the questions our children pose, fully relaxed. We should have the answers—about everything in and around sex, about stimulating aids, exciting variations, true love, intimacy, and well-intentioned advice.

Everyday Seduction

"HAROLD AND ANDREA, how are you?" I greet the couple for their last session for the time being. "Andrea wrote to me saying you might need a bit of inspiration on the topic of seduction." Both nod, and I have an idea.

When time allows, I work on an erotic card game intended to bring couples closer together physically. My card game is nearing completion and I want Harold and Andrea to try it out for me. They can be my guinea pigs.

My original reason for dreaming up the game was that clients, rather like Harold and Andrea, often said that they couldn't find the right moment to seduce their partners, and that they missed having something solid in their hands to make this easier—homework related to the therapy, or maybe some game or other? So on went the thinking cap. What kind of help could I provide these people? Games already on the market with names like "Erotic Dreams" or "Sexiness" mostly set a pretty swift pace; the right mood hardly has a chance to grow, let alone the desire to seduce. I must confess I don't like them. Who wants to draw a card only a few minutes after the game has started on which is written that they have to give their partner a blow job or vice versa? Much too direct, and not erotic at all. I felt these things should be a bit more leisurely, but how? In the end I just thought, *Okay. If there's nothing suitable to buy, I'll have to produce it myself.*

No sooner said than done. My own playing cards show erotic illustration of couples drawn by my present partner, Louis. He drew feet, hips, bosoms, butts, backs, mouths, and faces (full on and detailed). The game begins by getting to know each other better, and learning how to be intimate fully, not only with their bodies. The aim of the game is, first, for both players to tune in to their partner and then, later, to rustle up a slight sizzle of lust. At the beginning of the game, you ask questions like "If you were to change one thing about your childhood, what would it be?" and "What new skill would you like to wake up with tomorrow?" And last but not least, "What would you say to your father (or mother) if you knew you only had five days to live?" Questions like these seem, at first glance, to be puzzling and not particularly erotic. But the interesting thing about the questions, assuming people are being honest, is that vulnerability and intimacy can emerge from them. We learn something about our partner and ourselves. For those who think that questions like these would lead to quarrels, time is restricted: each question has to be answered within one minute.

In later stages of the game, sexual contact and seduction are introduced. Each player gets pleasure from achieving various small erotic "actions," this time for a minute, no longer! This raises the excitement level, makes you greedy for more—makes you feel that one minute was much too short. While you're playing, it's important to allow feelings to flow and to enjoy it. Pretty soon the game will be over— at least the card game!

Andrea and Harold are keen on the idea of being my game testers and eagerly look forward to telling me about whether it worked. We then go on to talk about other tips and tricks to bring a bit of zest to sex.

"You should go to one of my friend's workshops, craft classes," I say. Andrea looks a bit skeptical. Harold grins— I already told him about the courses during an individual session.

"Yes, Susanne Schülz goes through the various gripping techniques for the male and female genitalia," he expands.

"Do people touch each other?" Andrea is still a little doubtful.

"No," I say, "silicon models are used to illustrate various techniques. The classes are funny, and it's an exchange among adults." The courses are certainly recommended if you want to enhance your sexual confidence (Perception Sphere). You lose inhibitions, gain courage, and encourage creativity.

Andrea is obviously remembering the penis model that sat so easily in the hand and that she first encountered in my office, because she blushes when she notices that Harold is looking at her as if he can read her thoughts. But I have awakened her interest, because she asks when the next set of classes is to begin.

"We could try out the gripping techniques on each other," gushes Harold after noting down the dates. "And I can finally discover what you like—and we mustn't forget the oils." We have talked about various lubes and gels that can be used when masturbating.

"You could just use almond oil and cucumbers or carrots as dildos—there are no limits to inventiveness." I glance at Andrea and she immediately catches on. Perfect mind mapping! At the same time I try to map Harold. Has he already heard the cold carrot story? It doesn't seem so. As I suggested, Andrea seems to have kept some things to herself.

"What's up with you two?" Harold then asks. He's read both of us well and wants to be included.

Andrea replies coyly, "You don't have to know everything!" She seems to be enjoying flirting.

"What do you think about sexy underwear, Harold?" I ask.

"Oh, great!" he answers, a bit flummoxed.

"That's good, then Andrea can get some."

"She never wanted to wear them, so I guess something has really improved." Harold is visibly content.

I smile. "I meant sexy underwear for *you* to wear." Now I've caught him off guard. "The main thing is that the shorts hint at what's inside them and that the owner is aware of this." Andrea shows her endorsement with a cautious little nod. "Many men haven't discovered sexy underwear. So ditch the pack of three from the supermarket. Men can play with their sexual aura too. A six-pack is neither here nor there—we women don't look only at stomachs!"

Harold looks pensive.

Little Pink Pills

THERE ARE PLENTY of sex toys, many accessories, and umpteen gimmicks that can spark the libido or improve sex. Sexologists used to proclaim, "Sex toys, sex toys! Reinvent yourselves!" Since then the mood has shifted somewhat: "Be careful of vibrators!" Everything that buzzes and vibrates should be treated cautiously, as the body can quickly adapt to their use. You may have problems with your partner because, generally, the penis neither buzzes nor vibrates. It functions quite well without electric motors. Instead you might try lubes for smooth intercourse (they can be scented to smell of strawberries or lemons or, of course, be neutral). Or chili-based lubes—good for the circulation. Or how about some erotic literature, reading passages to each other? All of these can enrich and inspire. Additionally, there are artificial vaginas (fleshlights) and penises, inflatable anal plugs, cock rings, funny tongue tinglers, and dual-stimulating sex toys with or without remotes—each to his or her own.

If malfunctions in bed are to be avoided, auxiliary aids can sometimes make all the difference. Thus, for many people with sexual problems, the simple solution is to take a pill (swallow and go!). Drugs like Viagra and Cialis (sildena-fil and tadalafil) have been available for men for some time now. Unfortunately, they don't always work. The blue pills improve circulation in the penis (Physiological Sphere), but they perform their duties only when people are already aroused (Perception Sphere).

There is also a drive pill for women on the market, often called "pink Viagra," but it doesn't work in exactly the same way as the blue pill for men. The blue pill is taken only if someone is expecting to have sex in the very near future and is worried that without help he may suffer from embar-rassing limpness. Pink Viagra, on the other hand, has to be taken daily regardless of whether sex is on the agenda or not. I'm not a fan of the pink pills. Their side effects include fatigue, nausea, and dizziness, as well anything from low blood pressure right up to blackouts. Doesn't sound like much fun for foreplay, does it? Snoozing schmoozing! According to information from the U.S. regulatory author-ity, the side effects can be drastically aggravated when the pill is taken in conjunction with alcohol or tranquilizers. Additionally, people are warned against taking them during the day, as they can affect perception, such as when driving. Anyway, apart from all that, do they really work? According to a study by the manufacturer, women had satisfying sex 2.7 times a month without the pill and with the pill the figure increased to 4.4 times. But wait a sec! The result is misleading, as the test subjects who instead of taking the pink pill took a placebo, a sugar pill, had satisfying sex 3.7 times a month. This meant a paltry 0.7 times more sexu-ally gratifying events per month for the women taking the real pink Viagra, but also all the side effects. All I can say is, gimme the sugar pill! This shows that positive thoughts and feelings also have a lot of power in sexuality!

Homework without Side Effects

MY AUXILIARY AIDS contain no chemical components and thus don't have any side effects—except ones that are good and intended. By "auxiliary aids" I mean the refined and individually tuned homework that I give my clients. These aids have to be specific and manageable so that they stick in the brain. An example: Bridget had panic attacks every evening when she was preparing supper in the kitchen and heard her husband, Oliver, coming home, knowing that he would come to her and touch her. Bridget loved her husband but didn't like him greeting her like that. She felt a real aversion. So when she heard his footsteps, she stayed in the kitchen with her back to the door. When Oliver hugged her from behind, she reacted dismissively—almost aggressively. He was, of course, disappointed, and later became worried that something was fundamentally wrong with her. In discussions we discovered what the situation was like for Bridget, what triggered it, and the thoughts that automatically went through her head. To do this I used what is called a *cognitive protocol*. This involves writing down precisely how this automatism proceeds. After that, we develop a new reaction that should be practiced as a kind of homework. In this case, the protocol revealed that when her husband came home, Bridget's thoughts and feelings flashed back to scenes that she experienced when working for a few years as a prostitute in a brothel. Oliver had been one of her johns. She had a similar problem when workmen rang her doorbell. In both cases what was behind her actions was the belief that when a man came to her, she had to be friendly and do what he wanted. Bridget could, at some point, have told her husband, "I don't know why, but I have trouble when you come through the door. Could we talk about it?" But instead of talking about it, she had developed an aversion to her husband.

The homework for the couple now consisted of finding a different welcoming routine. As both had a good sense of humor, they thought it a good idea that Oliver crawl into the kitchen as if he were in an action movie. Bridget didn't like the other suggestion of Oliver waiting at the threshold and her going to the door to welcome him in (it reminded her too much of former situations). So action movie it was to be, and it worked. After five such welcomes, Bridget's early warning system settled down a bit and the danger was averted. She no longer became scared stiff when her husband came home—on the contrary, she looked forward to seeing her action hero!

Electric Toothbrushes and Other Oddments

RECENTLY I WAS in a bar with four girlfriends. We hadn't seen each other for a while and were catching up on news. At some stage (surprise, surprise!) the topic turned to sex. I told them about women who masturbated using electric toothbrushes. When the first client reported this, I was astonished; by the fourth or fifth, I had become hardened. It turned out, with a chorus of giggles, that my friends too had used electric toothbrushes for purposes not associated with dental hygiene. I was the only one who hadn't!

The fact is that people will go to all sorts of ends to arouse themselves, and can become pretty creative along the way. Sadly, sometimes things can go wrong. Vacuum cleaners, for instance, are well known not only for arousal but sometimes also for unexpected events. In the olden days there used to be a small fan built into the nozzle. People who stuck their penises into it, and apparently it wasn't just a few, seldom had ecstatic moments and were more likely to be the unwilling recipients of a circumcision—without medical assistance! The subsequent hospital stay must have been all the more embarrassing. The only things that can help at a time like that are a good dollop of humor and a marked sense of sexual self-confidence (Perception Sphere). Luckily, those propeller-based vacuum cleaners are now banned.

Astonishingly, many clients in their younger days used to do rhythmic pull-ups on their bedroom doorframes to get their kicks. Others simply dropped their pants and crawled under their beds to fumble about. One client used to rub dried stinging nettles up and down the shaft of his penis. Pretty resourceful! Luckily, he lived near the woods, so he had a good supply. Incidentally, he highly recommended *his* methods, but I'm not so sure. And speaking of woods, one client used to climb trees and dangle her legs on either side of a branch. She simply sat there and swayed. A natural? Somehow we all are.

Five Things I Want to Share with All Couples

1. **HANDS OFF NIPPLES!**

Nicole was an attractive physiotherapist, her husband a hospital janitor. She looked a little like Lady Di, the Princess of Hearts, with heavily lined eyes that were often downcast when she was talking to me. After ten years of marriage she was highly dissatisfied about how her husband approached her when he wanted sex. Without any signs of tenderness, he just made a grab for her nipples, something she didn't like anyway. She was furious when he started groping her nipples, but unfortunately only inwardly. When I asked her why she played along with him without objecting, she explained, eyes downcast again, that she didn't dare tell him. How often have I heard something similar! Men, believe us: most women don't feel like sex when you start twisting our nipples. The fact is that women only begin to enjoy being stimulated there after they're already aroused. My advice to all women is say something immediately, and certainly don't try to hide your displeasure.

2. **BE YOURSELF!**

People tend to measure themselves against an ideal even though a comparison to the average would be more suitable. Better still, don't compare yourself to anyone. After all, you are unique!

3. **BE CURIOUS**

You have to have sex—everyone says so. Statistically, apparently, 2.6 times a week, although in long-term relationships with children and all, this is completely unrealistic. Sex is not a drive like it was thought to be for a long time. The deeply anchored belief that men are creatures driven by lust and women are seductresses implies that men have a natural claim or even right to sex. Conveniently (for men), women often take others' needs more seriously than their own. This pressure-cooker model—instinctive needs have to be satisfied or things will explode—is now considered out of date. If sex isn't a drive, then, how *does* it work? Experts speak of *incentive motivation,* in which we want to have sex because we expect positive consequences. You could say that sexual desire is rather like curiosity. So be curious, about your partner and about life!

4. SCREENS OFF!

The digital world has captured us. It shapes our relationships, and not always for the good of all. Pressures and dissatisfaction are on the increase, personal happiness declining. My advice: Put electronic devices like cellphones and tablets aside. Better yet, turn them right off. In general, try to slow down. This also applies in the bedroom! Shut down electronic devices, at least once a week. How about it?

5. LOVE IS ... STOPPING FOR A BREAK

What we mustn't forget in all this is love. I am often asked, "What do you think of as love?" My answer is always prompt: "It's the small, short moments of happiness."

When I got to know my partner Louis, I was in a daze. It was not my new companion that triggered this but my work. I had just published my first book, and I felt as if everyone wanted something from me. With all the questions coming in, try as I might, I couldn't pull on the handbrake. Louis looked on, worried; it seemed almost like our relationship was going to end before it even got properly started. I was not only short-winded but short-tempered. I was pure stress! He couldn't stop me. Then, at the last moment, he stepped in and dared to say something: "You can't carry on like this, honey. You need some peace and quiet!"

Yes, I needed peace and quiet, and in one sentence, at exactly the right time, Louis had given me the nudge I needed. What sounds so easy was difficult, but in the end it succeeded. Wherever possible, I withdrew. I became more mindful of myself and my time. Afterward I was back again but different. I had reshuffled the cards. Every day I kiss the man who told me to take a break, with his worries about me and his typically mild look. This is love, for me!

A Happy Ending

ANDREA AND HAROLD—I haven't forgotten them. Since their first session in my office, they have both come a long way. Andrea can now have orgasms; Harold's erections have been stabilized. Nowadays he masturbates when he feels like it, and my impression is that Andrea does too. She has relaxed and now talks easily about sex. New underwear has been bought, and both practice seduction playfully. The playing cards were a success: the questions in particular inspired them and helped them experience intimacy.

Andrea and Harold wanted more intimacy in their daily routine. If a couple manage to create intimacy, wonderful things can happen. I often experience it with Louis. We sit there talking intently—in full daylight, mind you—and suddenly I say, "Oh, what was that? I was so close to you and all of a sudden I have an urge to touch you." If there *is* a magic trick to passion and love, it is intimacy. It's an extremely powerful tool that is completely underestimated by many people. But what exactly is intimacy?

Intimacy means transparency, communication, openness, shared feelings as well as shared experiences (and not only the good ones!). Truth comes to light as if under a microscope, particularly things associated with fear, so that the partner can know about them. Making these truths visible is necessary and unburdening, because holding something back costs energy and keeps couples apart even though they are together. It requires a lot of strength to back away from a partner, to shut yourself off from somebody so they can't read what's rumbling inside you. The other party then also withdraws, and already you find them less attractive. After all, they're no longer really on your side. Both partners retreat inside their respective shells—a vicious circle in which many people are stuck.

Intimacy is all about sharing real feelings, thoughts, and needs with someone close to you, someone who wishes to *remain* close to you and become even closer. Intimacy relieves pressure and at the same time is sexy.

The wonderful thing is that, at any point in time, couples together in intimate, close contact can also lead lively sex lives.

That is how it is for Andrea and Harold. If they continue to be honest with each other and are able to accept glitches and occasional rebuffs without becoming frightened, then they might make a success of their relationship. And I tell them just that.

During the final session with them, I receive one last piece of information: "Our dog, Tussie, died last Friday. We looked for a breeder right away, and in two weeks we'll get a puppy." I wanted to ask about its sex when both proclaimed in unison: "She's called Lassie!" They looked at each other in surprise, laughed, and Andrea screamed: "Oh no! A symbiotic relapse!"

And even if it was, as long as they're aware of it, all is well.

Departures

I WAS ON the train. It was summer but rainy and cold. I was wearing light clothes since when I'd caught the train, the sun, for once, had been shining in Hamburg. Annoyed, I looked through the steamed-up window into the gloom. The train's departure had been delayed for almost twenty minutes. Half an hour later, I was stranded in another station as my connecting train pulled out of the station right in front of my eyes.

Shivering, I looked around. The station was being renovated but there was a temporary information service operating from a small booth on the platform. What seemed like hours ago now, I was supposed to have given a telephone interview on the topic of orgasms, but reception in the train had been bad and the connection kept breaking down. Very annoying, the whole situation, but probably not for all passengers. After all, not everyone wants to be reminded about orgasms on a train journey. I can whisper as much as I like, but a few people always pick up on the conversation.

In front of the information booth, I considered the possibility of continuing the phone interview. My feet were cold in my leather flip-flops, so I went into the little booth. Inside were five railway officials, four women and a man, but no other passengers, which prompted me to ask the people in uniform (admittedly a little too loudly), "Excuse me, do you think it would be possible for me to conduct a telephone interview here on female genitalia—including orgasms?"

Five pairs of wide-open eyes stared at me.

"It's just that there doesn't seem to be anybody...apart from you, of course..."

Silence. I tried to discover whether my enquiry was too much for these good souls. Then suddenly a bright voice broke the silence. One of the female railway officials exclaimed cheerfully, "Oh, Ms. Henning! Of course!" The nice lady led me up a narrow staircase to a little break room. I was brought a coffee and some milk and was able to complete the interview...with one interruption—the friendly railway woman cautiously popped her head in and held up a sheet of paper informing me that my train was delayed. By nine minutes, to be exact. Now nobody can tell me that the railway doesn't offer good service! The moral of the story is this: under certain circumstances, whoever floats a question about sex in a room will have pleasantly warm feet not long after. *Let's talk about sex.*

Acknowledgments

I'D LIKE TO thank many people, beginning with Louis Harrison, my partner, my companion, who, as he says, has a never-ending belief in my powers, my stamina, and my intelligence.

Regina Carstensen assisted me so superbly, inspired me to write, and effortlessly improved my mood with her warm laughter when things seemed too gloomy.

Barbara Laugwitz has a pretty good idea of how "Ann-Marlene's voice" should sound and kept doing the rounds until this "voice" was present in the manuscript.

My friends don't even know how good it is of them to put up with my postponing or canceling our meetings when I'm working on a book. They don't reproach me; they simply love me just as much after the book as before.

Gunnar Henriksen, my grandpa, taught me early to persevere and to finish doing anything that I started—without those lessons, this book wouldn't have existed.

About the Author

ANN-MARLENE HENNING IS a sexologist and couples therapist practicing in Hamburg, Germany. Born and raised in Denmark, she moved to Germany in 1985. She studied neuropsychology at the University of Hamburg while working as a model before returning to Denmark to study sexology. She then continued her education at the Zurich Institute for Clinical Sexology and Sexual Therapy, and recently completed her Masters in sexology at the Merseburg College of Applied Sciences. In her practice, she helps her clients develop healthy relationships with both their partners and their own sexuality.

She has published six books, including *Make Love*, which was nominated for the German Youth Literature Award in 2013, and *Make More Love*. She demystifies sex therapy in her video blog *Doch Noch*, and hosts the popular TV documentary series, also called *Make Love*, which was nominated for the German Television Award in 2017. Besides her writing and television work, she has also created an erotic-therapeutic card game.

Ann-Marlene has one son and lives with her partner in Hamburg.